Third Edition

Review in Pathology with Colour Plates

STUDENTS' COMPANION

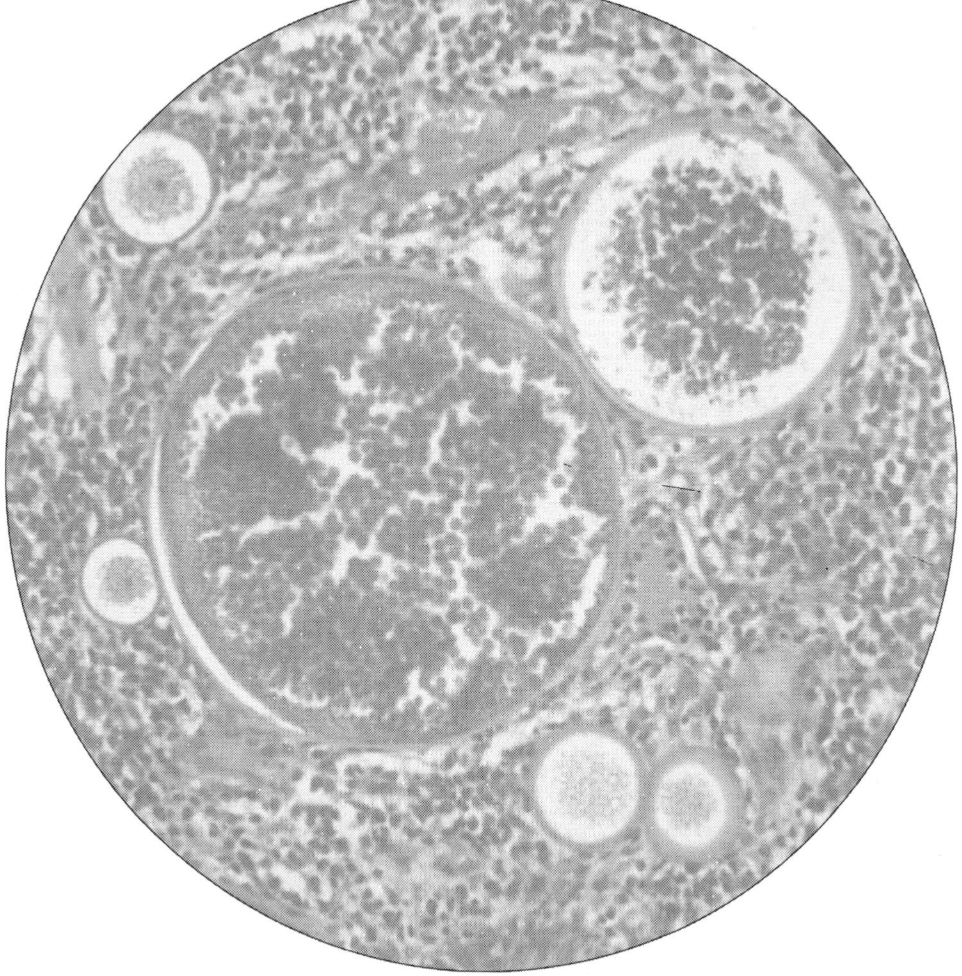

Third Edition

Review in Pathology with Colour Plates

STUDENTS' COMPANION

Nitiin Chaawla MBBS, FAGE, MD (Pathology), PGDHA, MBA (HCM)
Deputy Chief Medical Officer
Department of Pathology
SP Wahi Hospital
ONGC (Oil and Natural Gas Corporation) Ltd.
Dehradun, Uttarakhand, India

Sandip Kudesia MBBS, MD (Pathology), PhD (Neuropathology), FAIMER
Professor, Department of Pathology
Sohar Medical College, Oman

CBSPD

CBS Publishers & Distributors Pvt Ltd

New Delhi • Bengaluru • Chennai • Kochi • Kolkata • Lucknow • Mumbai
Hyderabad • Jharkhand • Nagpur • Patna • Pune • Uttarakhand

Third Edition
Review in
Pathology with Colour Plates
STUDENTS' COMPANION

ISBN: 978-93-5466-062-7

Third Edition: 2022
Reprint: 2024, 2025
First Edition: 2012
Second Edition: 2018
Reprint: 2019

Published by Satish Kumar Jain and produced by Varun Jain for

CBS Publishers & Distributors Pvt Ltd
4819/XI Prahlad Street, 24 Ansari Road, Daryaganj, New Delhi 110 002, India
Ph: 011-23289259, 23266838 Website: www.cbspd.com
e-mail: delhi@cbspd.com
Corporate Office: 204 FIE, Industrial Area, Patparganj, Delhi 110 092
Ph: 011-4934 4934 Fax: 011-4934 4935 e-mail: publishing@cbspd.com; publicity@cbspd.com

Branches

- **Bengaluru:** Seema House 2975, 17th Cross, K.R. Road, Banasankari 2nd Stage, Bengaluru 560 070, Karnataka, India
  Ph: +91-80-26771678/79 Fax: +91-80-26771680 e-mail: bangalore@cbspd.com
- **Chennai:** 18/8B, Subbarayan Street, Shenoy Nagar, Chennai 600 030, Tamil Nadu, India
  Ph: +91-44-42032115, 26681266 e-mail: chennai@cbspd.com
- **Kochi:** 42/1325, 1326, Power House Road, Opp KSEB, Power House, Ernakulam 682 018, Kerala, India
  Ph: +91-484-4059061-65 Fax: +91-484-4059065 e-mail: kochi@cbspd.com
- **Kolkata:** 147, Hind Ceramics Compound, 1st Floor, Nilgunj Road, Belghoria, Kolkata-700056, West Bengal, India
  Ph: 033-25633055, 033-25633056 e-mail: kolkata@cbspd.com
- **Lucknow:** Basement, Khushnuma Complex, 7-Meerabai Marg (Behind Jawahar Bhawan), Lucknow 226001, India
  Ph: 0522-4000032 e-mail: tiwari.lucknow@cbspd.com
- **Mumbai:** PWD Shed. Gala no. 25/26, Ramchandra Bhatt Marg, Next to JJ Hospital Gate no. 2 Opp. Union Bank of India Noorbaug Mumbai-400009, Maharashtra, India
  Ph: 022-66661880/89 e-mail: mumbai@cbspd.com

Representatives

- **Hyderabad** 0-9885175004 • **Jharkhand** 0-9811541605 • **Nagpur** 0-8692091830
- **Patna** 0-9334159340 • **Pune** 0-9664372571 • **Uttarakhand** 0-9716462459

Printed at Rashtriya Printers, Delhi, India

Disclaimer

Preface to the Third Edition

Three years back we had come up with the second edition of the book. Continued support from the medical students has led us to come up with a revised edition. The students have loved this book which has given us the desired mojo to create this edition. Few new topics have been added based on the recent advances and few coloured plates of pictures have been added. Though this is a review book but students have time and again made us realize that this book is their true companion in understanding the subject of pathology as well as helped them in passing their exams with extraordinary results.

We thankfully acknowledge the kind support our both the volumes have received from the medical students and teachers of various medical colleges across the globe.

We would like to thank Mr YN Arjuna and his entire publishing team who have constantly supported us unflinchingly in successful revision of every new edition of the book.

Nitiin Chaawla
Sandip Kudesia

All figures cited in the text are given in **Colour Plates 1–18** inserted between pages 8 and 9.

Preface to the First Edition

This handbook was conceptualized based on our own experiences in undergraduate days when such material was collected from different sources, including lecture notes made during classes and noted down in the corners of standard textbooks for easy and quick revision prior to examinations.

This compilation of data is tailor-made for undergraduate students of pathology who have read standard textbooks on the subject to help them revise and recollect important topics in a relatively short time from examination point of view. All relevant information has been grouped into flowcharts for easier visual association. It is also meant to be a helpful revision companion for those aspiring of getting admission through PG entrance examinations.

Based on MCI approved syllabus, the book covers 134 topics considered relevant and important contextually. Students may wish to read the chapters in sequence, or as per their curriculum requires. This manual is not a substitute to the standard textbooks on pathology but will serve as a 'companion' to the student making it easier to assimilate and recall by presenting the subject matter in the form of flowcharts containing easy to remember points on the topics.

This is the first-ever book in presenting the subject of pathology topic-wise in an easy-to-read and recall student-friendly format. We may say that we have laboured long and earnestly to prepare this text so that it becomes a firm and helpful guide to the students.

We earnestly request the students and teachers to communicate any suggestions which may tend to improve this book in its second edition; whatever can be done to make this book of greater service to the medical students will be gladly undertaken.

Nitiin Chaawla
Sandip Kudesia

Acknowledgements

We thank our honorable chairman of SGRR education mission Mahant Shri Devendra Dass ji Maharaj for his vision and his constant motivation towards all creative and constructive socially useful endeavours.

We thank Dr. Sanjeev Kishore, Professor, Department of Pathology, for his useful support in compilation of this work.

We thank Mr Amit Thaledi, laboratory technician and computer operator of our department, for his meticulous and quick compilation of our work.

Above all we thank the Almighty who gave us the ability and perseverance to compile this book.

Nitiin Chaawla
Sandip Kudesia

Contents

CELLULAR ADAPTATIONS

Definition: They are defined as adaptive changes taking place in a tissue or an organ secondary to altered physiological stimulation.

Causes
- Increased demand
- Increased hormonal stimulation
- Decreased nutrients
- Chronic physical or chemical irritation.

Types

Hyperplasia
- **Definition:** It is defined as an increase in number of cells in a tissue or an organ leading to increase in its size.
- **Types**
  - Physiological hyperplasia—e.g. hyperplasia of breast ducts and lobules during puberty and lactation, hyperplasia of uterus during pregnancy
  - Pathological hyperplasia—e.g. benign prostatic hyperplasia **(Fig. 42)**, endometrial hyperplasia. **(Fig. 47)**

Metaplasia
- **Definition:** It is defined as reversible transformation of one cell type into another cell type secondary to chronic irritation.
- **Types**
  - Columnar to squamous metaplasia, e.g. bronchial epithelium due to chronic irritants present an cigarette smoke
  - Squamous to columnar metaplasia, e.g. Barret esophagus **(Fig. 1)**
  - Connective tissue metaplasia, e.g. Myositis ossificans.

Hypertrophy
- **Definition:** It is defined as an increase in size of cells in a tissue or an organ leading to increase in its size.
- **Types**
  - Physiological hypertrophy—e.g. hypertrophy of skeletal muscles due to repetitive workouts in gymnasium
  - Pathological hypertrophy—e.g. left ventricular hypertrophy due to systemic circulation overload.

Atrophy
- **Definition:** It is defined as shrinkage in size of cells by loss of intracellular organelles leading to shrinkage of organ.
- **Types (based on cause)**
  - Disuse atrophy—e.g. skeletal muscle atrophy secondary to immobilization in cast following fracture
  - Denervation atrophy—e.g. atrophy of muscle secondary to nerve injury supplying it
  - Ischemic atrophy—Atrophy of an organ secondary to diminished blood supply
  - Nutritional atrophy—e.g. atrophy of skeletal muscles due to protein energy malnutrition
  - Senile atrophy—e.g. atrophy of breast after menopause
  - Endocrinal atrophy–e.g. atrophy of uterus and breast after menopause
  - Pressure atrophy—e. g. A tumor compresses the surrounding organ causing its shrinkage.

CELL INJURY

Types

Reversible cell injury

- Morphological changes seen are:
  - Cell membrane bleb formation
  - Swelling of endoplasmic reticulum and mitochondria
  - Clumping of nuclear chromatin.

Irreversible cell injury

- Morphological changes seen are:
  - Large cell membrane blebs
  - Swelling of endoplasmic reticulum and loss of ribosomes
  - Rupture of lysosomes
  - Swelling of mitochondria with formation of amorphous densities
  - Myelin figures formed under cell membrane
  - Nuclear condensation.

Causes

- Hypoxia
- Infectious agents
- Physical agents
- Drugs and chemicals
- Immunological reactions
- Genetic derangements
- Nutritional imbalances.

Mechanisms

Accamalation of O_2 derived free radicals

- Free radicals are accumulated due to imbalance between free radical producing and free radical scavenger mechanisms
- The free radicals cause cell damage by lipid peroxidation of membranes, oxidation of proteins and by producing lesions in DNA.

Increased intracellular calcium

- Loss of sodium pump and mitochondrial injury leads to elevation of intracellular calcium ion levels causing activation of various enzymes like ATPase, phospholipase, protease, endonuclease which leads to degradation of cytoplasmic organelles and nuclear material.

Mitochondrial damage: Damage to mitochondria leads to:

- Exodus of cytochrome C and hydrogen ions into the cytoplasm which leads to initiation of apoptosis.

Decrease in ATP: Depleted ATP leads to:

- Decreased sodium pump activity leading to increased intracellular sodium, calcium ions and water causing cell and endoplasmic reticulum swelling
- Increase anaerobic glycolysis causing lactic acidosis leading to nuclear chromatin clumping
- Detachment of ribosomes inhibiting protein production.

NECROSIS

Definition: It is defined as the morphological changes taking place in a tissue after cell death due to degradative action of enzymes on irreversibly injured cell.

Morphological changes

Cytoplasmic changes
- Increased eisonophilia of cytoplasm
- Vacuolation and moth eaten appearance of cytoplasm
- Calcification of cell membrane and intracellular structures
- Formations of myelin figures.

Nuclear changes
- *Karyolysis*: Fading of basophilia of nucleus
- *Pyknosis*: Nuclear shrinkage due to condensation of chromatin
- *Karyorrhexis*: Nuclear fragmentation.

Types

Caseous necrosis
- It is seen in tuberculosis and occurs due to both enzymatic degradation of tissues and denaturation of cellular proteins
- The tissue architecture is lost and replaced by soft, creamy cheese like material **(Image B)**
- Microscopically, there is amorphous granular debris seen **(Fig. 4)**
- Example: Tuberculosis lymph node, tuberculosis lung.

Liquefactive necrosis
- It is caused by enzymatic degradation of tissue
- The tissue undergoing liquefactive necrosis undergoes softening with destruction of architecture and accumulation of semifluid pus
- The cellular outlines of cells in tissue are completely lost
- Examples: Cerebral abscess, spinal cord abscess.

Coagulative necrosis
- It is caused by denaturation of intracellular proteins
- The cellular out lines of necrosed tissue is maintained **(Fig. 2)**
- The organ undergoing coagulative necrosis have firm texture **(Image A)**
- Examples: Myocardial infarction, renal infarcts.

NECROSIS (contd.) → **Types (contd.)**

Fibrinoid necrosis (Fig. 5)

- It occurs in walls of blood vessels secondary to injury leading to insudation and accumulation of plasma proteins giving an eosinophilic hue
- Examples: Fibrinoid necrosis of blood vessel in immune and non-immune vasculitis.

Gangrenous necrosis

- It is coagulative necrosis of tissue with superadded putrefaction by putrefactive bacteria e.g. *Clostridium* species
- Grossly, the organ is grayish black in colour and foul smelling
- Examples: Intestinal gangrene, gangrene of fingers.

Fat necrosis

- It is seen in adipose tissue and is characterized by grey white chalky deposits in fatty tissue **(Image C)**
- Microscopically, shadowy outlines of necrotic adipocytes with foreign body giant cells and basophilic calcification deposits are seen **(Fig. 3)**
- **Types**
    - Traumatic fat necrosis seen in breast and buttocks following blunt trauma
    - Enzymatic fat necrosis seen in acute pancreatitis.

APOPTOSIS

Definition: It is a cell death pathway in which a cell which has to die secretes enzymes for degradation of its contents, i.e. organelles and nucleus.

Causes

Physiological apoptosis
- Destruction of cells during embryogenesis
- Hormone dependant involution of cells, e.g. endometrium at end of menstrual cycle
- Destruction of cells in proliferating tissue, e.g. intestinal epithelial cells
- Death of cells after usage, e.g. erythrocyte destruction after 120 days.

Pathological apoptosis
- Death of cells in tumors
- Cell death due to viral infections, e.g. hepatocytes in viral hepatitis B
- Atrophy of parenchymal organs, e.g. parotid gland atrophy secondary to duct obstruction.

Morphology

Ultrastructural changes
- Cell shrinkage
- Chromatin condensation
- Formation of cytoplasmic blebs.

Histological changes
- Single cell or cluster of cells are involved
- Formation of round or oval mass of eosinophilic cytoplasm with dense nuclear fragments are called apoptotic bodies
- No inflammation
- Quick phagocytosis of dead cells.

Mechanism

- It is divided into 2 phases:
  - *Initiation phase*: It occurs by 2 pathways:
    - Extrinsic pathway
    - Intrinsic pathways
  - *Execution phase*

Intrinsic (Mitochondrial) pathway
- Cells destined to die undergo alteration in mitochondrial permeability
- This alteration leads to release of cytochrome C from inner mitochondrial membrane into cytoplasm
- Cytochrome C binds with apoptosis activating factors leading to activation of caspase 9.

Extrinsic (Death receptor) pathway
- Engagement of cell surface death receptors on cells
- Death receptor have a Fas domain and cytoplasmic death domain
- Binding of Fas ligand to Fas leads to clustering of multiple death receptors forming. Fas associated death domain (FADD)
- FADD binds with procaspases 8 and 10 to form active caspases.

Execution phase
- Initiation caspases lead to activation of executioner caspases, i.e. caspase 6 and 3
- These executioner caspases act on cellular and nuclear proteins and cleave them after aspartic acid residues causing their degradation
- Dying cells secrete factors which induce macrophage phagocytosis.

PATHOLOGICAL CALCIFICATION

Definition: It is defined as the deposition of calcium salts with small amount of mineral salts in tissues **(Fig. 6)**.

Pathogenesis

- Pathogenetic process has 2 phases:
  1. *Initiation phase*: In this phase, phospholipid vesicles are formed and hydroxyapatite crystals are deposited in it.
  2. *Proliferation phase*: The amount of calcium and phosphate ions in serum determines the amount of hydroxyapatite deposited in the tissue.

Types

Metastatic calcification

- It occurs in normal living tissues.
- There is associated serum increased calcium levels
- It is seen in:
  - Hyperparathyroidism
  - Hyperthyroidism
  - Hypervitaminosis D
  - Addison disease
  - Metastatic tumors in bone
  - Renal failure.

Dystrophic calcification

- It is seen in necrosed or degenerating tissues.
  - Long-standing tuberculosis focus
  - Older cyst in breast or thyroid
  - Organized thrombus
  - Degenerating joint cartilages
  - Prolapsed intervertebral disc
  - Tunica media of uterine blood vessels
- It is associated with normal serum calcium levels.

INFLAMMATION

Definition: It is defined as a response to injurious agents that consist of vascular responses, migration and activation of leucocytes and phagocytosis.

Cardinal signs of inflammation

- Rubor (redness)
- Calor (heat)
- Dolor (pain)
- Tumor (swelling)
- Functio laesa (loss of function)

Causes

- Infectious organisms
- Trauma
- Immune reactions
- Physical agents
- Chemical agents
- Foreign bodies.

Components of inflammation

- Inflammatory process has 2 main components:
  - Vascular events
  - Cellular events

Types

Acute inflammation (Fig. 7 and Image D)

- Rapid onset (within minutes)
- Lasting for few days
- Exudation of plasma proteins
- Emigration of neutrophils.

Chronic inflammation (Fig. 8 and Image E)

- Longer duration
- Lasting for weeks to months
- Associated with accumulation of lymphocytes and histiocytes.

Subtypes (of acute inflammation)

Acute purulent inflammation

- Characterized by accumulation of pus composed of neutrophils, necrotic material and edema fluid, e.g. abscess.

Acute serous inflammation

- Characterized by accumulation of thin serous fluid, e.g. pleural effusion, skin vesicles and blisters.

Acute fibrinous inflammation

- Large particles of fibrinogen accumulate at site of inflammation which is seen microscopically as eosinophilic threads, e.g. pericarditis, pleuritis, meningitis.

VASCULAR EVENTS IN INFLAMMATION

Vasodilation
- First vascular event
- It follows transient period of vasoconstriction of arterioles.

Increased permeability of microvasculature
- Exudation is hall mark of acute inflammation
- It doesn't occur though normal vascular endothelium
- It occurs due to increased vascular permeability secondary to response against inciting cause.

Stasis of blood
- Third vascular event which occurs due to increased viscosity of blood as a result of fluid exudation
- It takes 15–30 minutes after inciting stimulus affection
- Stasis of blood leads to margination of leucocytes towards vascular endothelium.

Mechanisms of increased vascular permeability

Direct endothelial injury
- Seen in necrotizing injuries
- Affects capillaries, arterioles and venules
- Fast and long lived lasting hours to days.

Delayed prolonged leakage
- Begins 2–12 hours after injury and lasts for several hours to days
- Affect venules as well as capillaries
- Causes–Thermal injury, radiation injury.

Endothelial gap formation
- Most common
- Rapid and short-lived
- Affects venules 20–60 mm in size
- Mediators involved-histamine, leukotrienes, bradykinin

Leakage from new blood vessels
- Late response occur during repair
- Mediators involved–Histamine, substance P, vascular endothelial growth factor.
- VEGF

Leucocyte mediated endothelial injury
- Affects venules and capillaries
- Late response lasting hours to days
- Leucocytes adhere to endothelium and release tissue O_2 species which cause endothelial damage.

Increased transcytosis across endothelial cell cytoplasm
- It occurs along vesiculovacuolar channels located near intercellular junctions in venules
- Mediators involved-vascular endothelial growth factor.

Plate 1

Histopathology

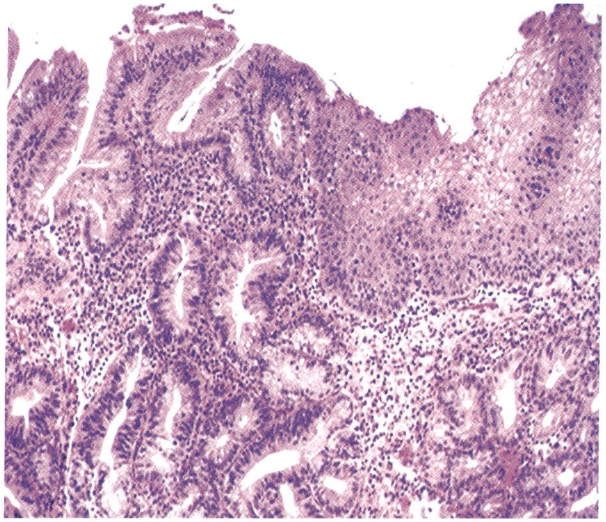

Figure 1: Squamous to columnar metaplasia—Photomicrograph showing columnar metaplasia of lower esophageal epithelium (left).

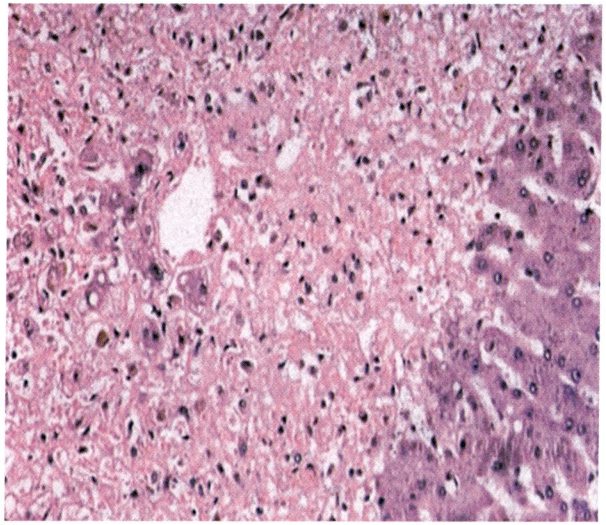

Figure 2: Coagulative necrosis—Photomicrograph displaying coagulative necrosis (Left) and normal hepatocytes (Right).

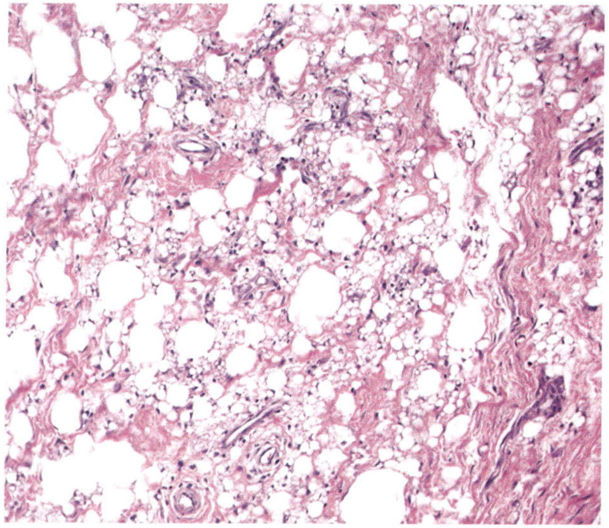

Figure 3: Fat necrosis—Photomicrograph displaying necrotic adipocytes mixed with inflammatory cells and foci of calcification.

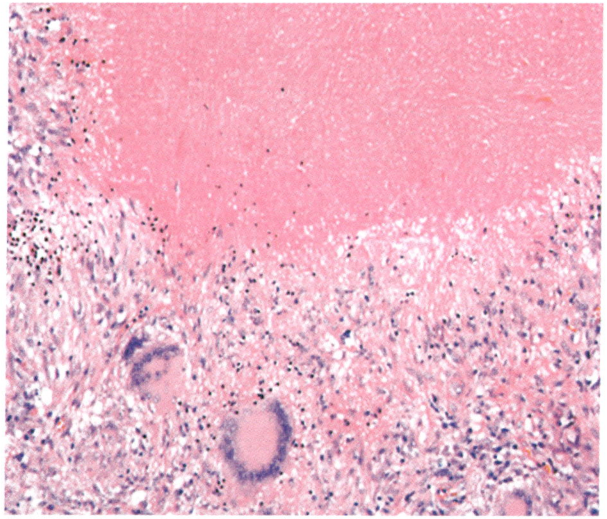

Figure 4: Caseous necrosis—Photomicrograph displaying caseous necrosis(top) with epithelioid granulomata and Langhans giant cells (Below).

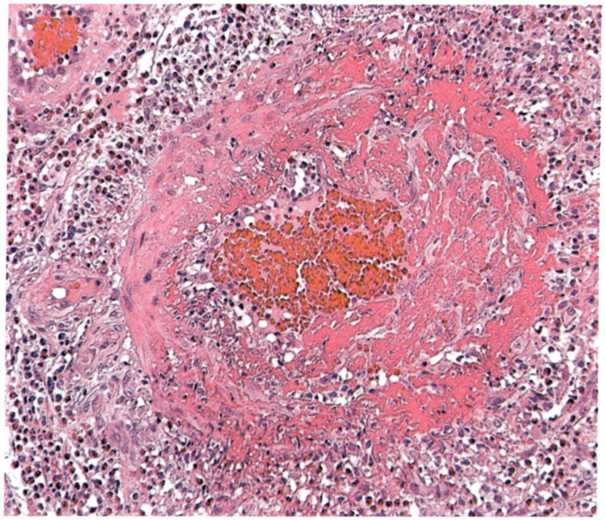

Figure 5: Fibrinoid necrosis—Photomicrograph displaying a thrombosed blood vessel with fibrinoid necrosis in its wall.

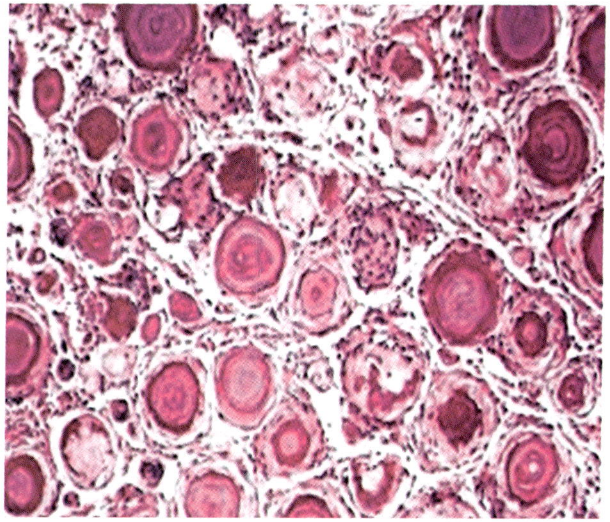

Figure 6: Pathological calcification—Photomicrograph displaying multiple basophilic lamellated calcification deposits also known *Psammoma bodies.*

Plate 2

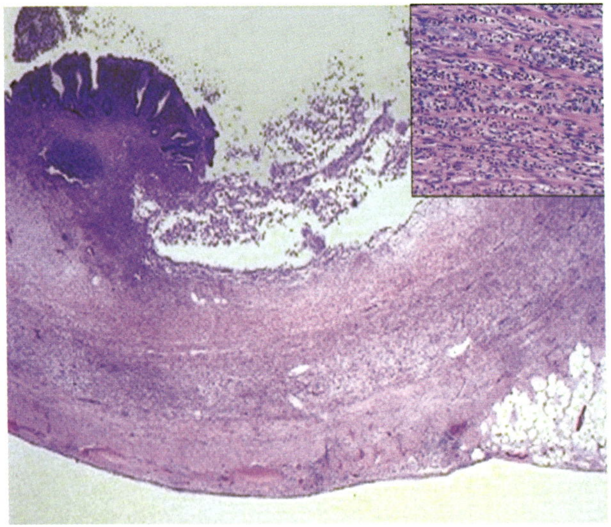

Figure 7: Acute appendicitis—Photomicrograph displaying luminal abscess, mucosal ulceration and neutrophilic infiltrate in submucosa, muscularis propria and serosa. Neutrophils seen in muscularis propria (Inset).

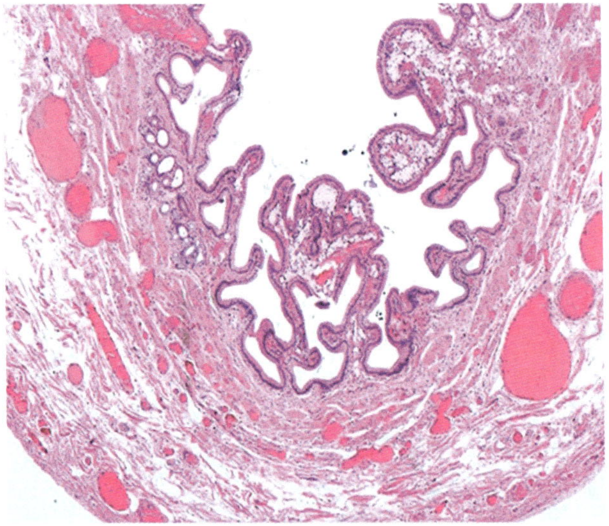

Figure 8: Chronic cholecystitis—Photomicrograph displaying infoldings of lining epithelium (Rokitansky-Aschoff sinus) with lymphohistiocytic infiltrate in submucosa. There are congested blood vessels and fibrosis seen in serosa.

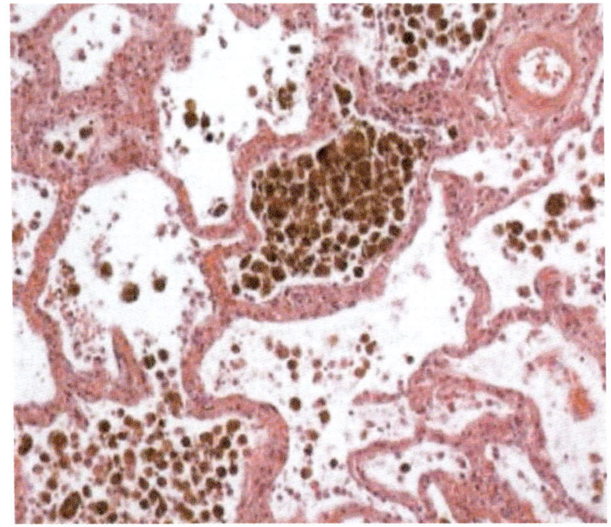

Figure 9: CVC Lung—Photomicrograph displaying thickened alveolar septae with hemosiderin laden macrophages within alveoli.

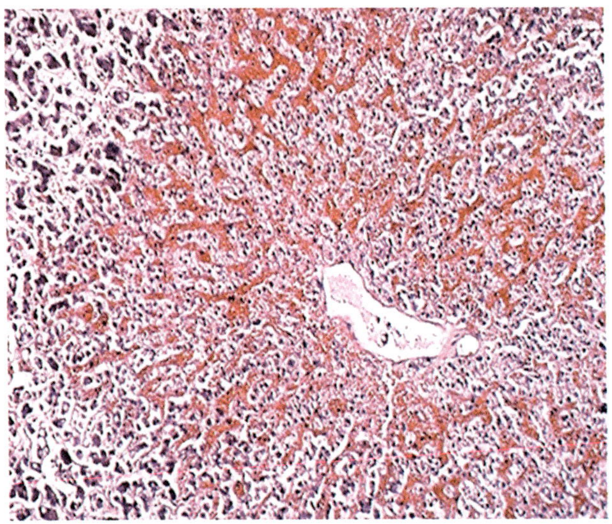

Figure 10: CVC Liver—Photomicrograph displaying dilated sinusoids filled with blood around the central vein with normal sinusoids away from it (Left).

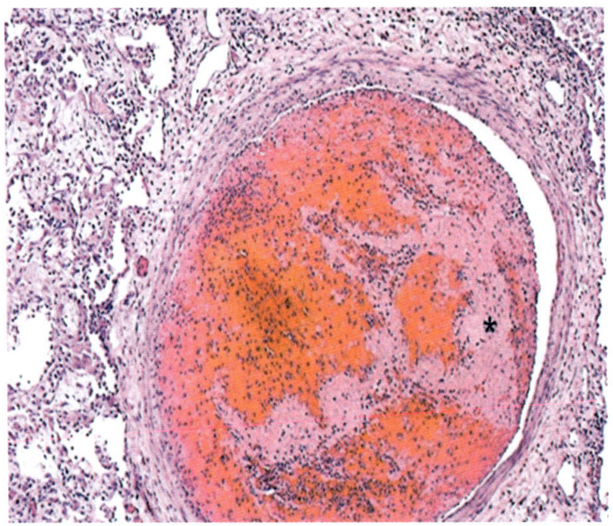

Figure 11: Thrombus—Photomicrograph displaying a dilated vein with a thrombus within it.

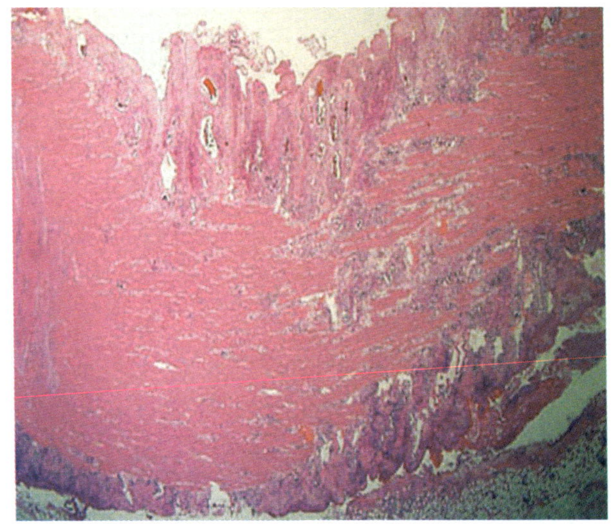

Figure 12: Infarct intestine—Photomicrograph displaying transmural hemorrhagic infarct in intestine.

Plate 3

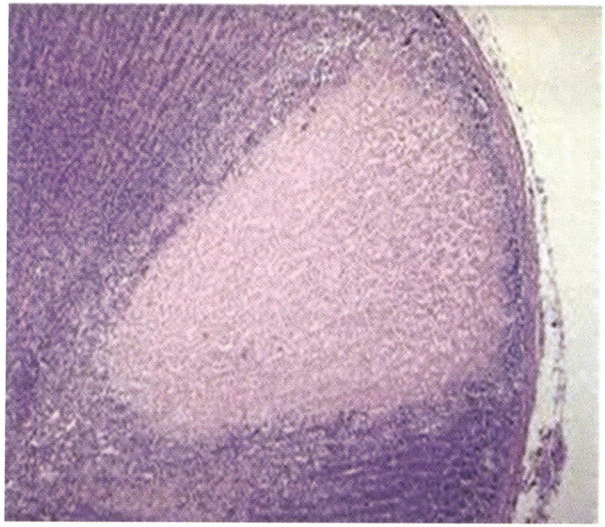

Figure 13: White infarct spleen—Photomicrograph displaying a well-defined white infarct in subcapsular region of spleen.

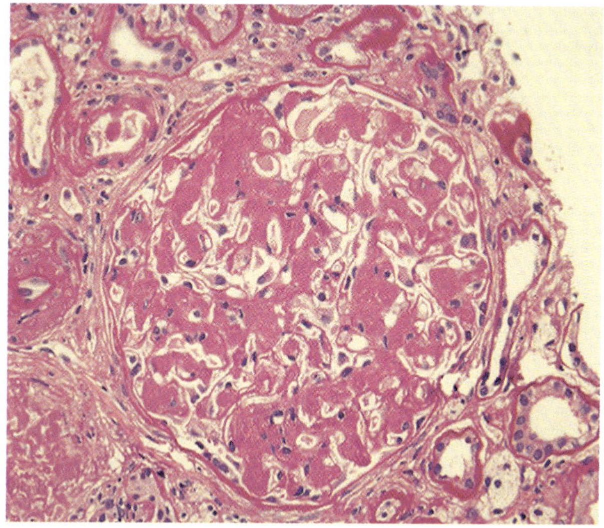

Figure 14: Renal amyloidosis—Photomicrograph displaying eosinophilic amyloid deposition in a renal glomerulus.

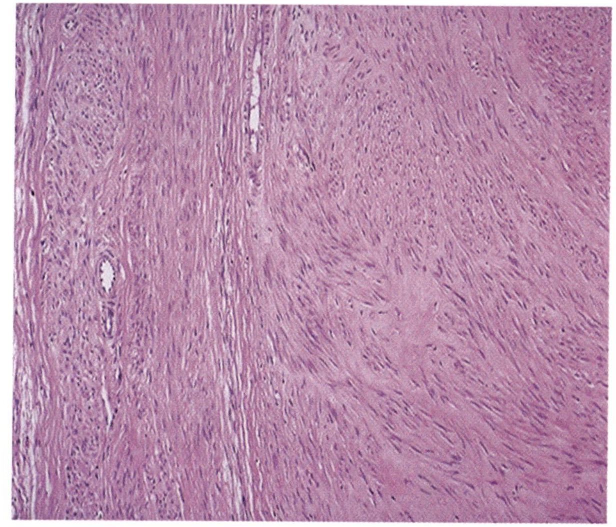

Figure 15: Leiomyoma—Photomicrograph displaying a benign tumor composed of interlacing fascicles of smooth muscle fibres.

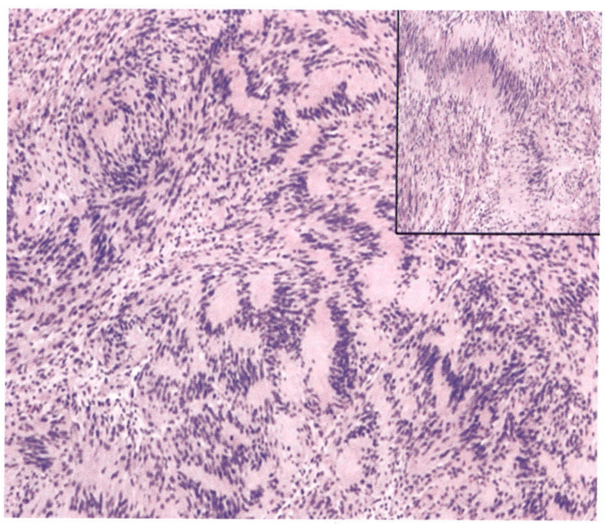

Figure 16: Neurilemmoma—Photomicrograph displaying a nerve sheath tumor composed of hypercellular (Antoni A) and hypocellular (Antoni B) areas with presence of verocay Bodies (Inset).

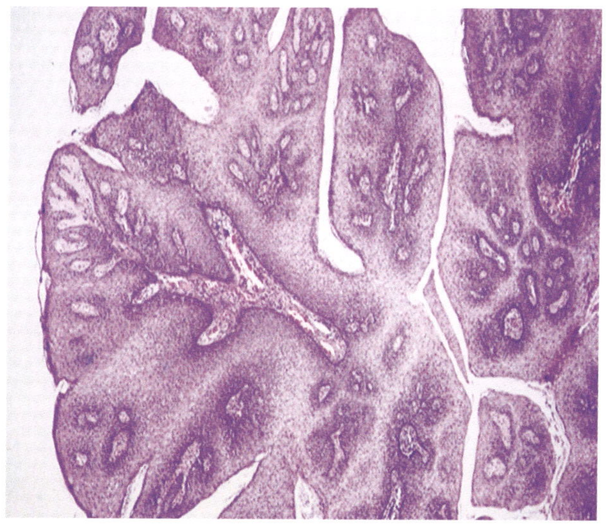

Figure 17: Squamous papilloma—Photomicrograph displaying a benign epithelial tumor showing papillar projections lined by hyperplastic stratified squamous epithelium.

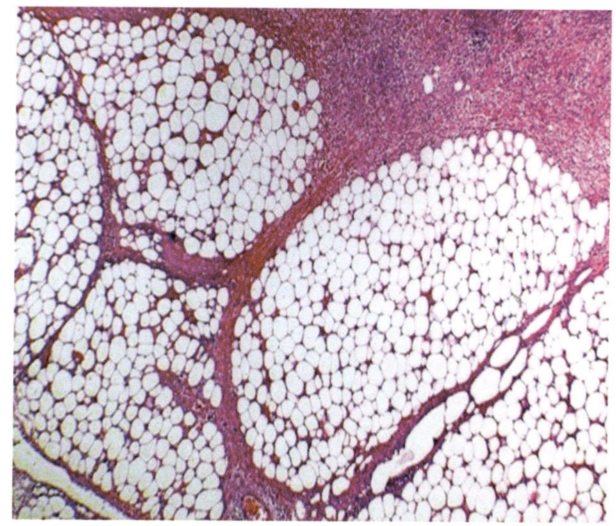

Figure 18: Lipoma—Photomicrograph displaying encapsulated benign well-circumscribed benign tumor composed of sheets of mature adipocytes with scanty intervening fibrous stroma.

Plate 4

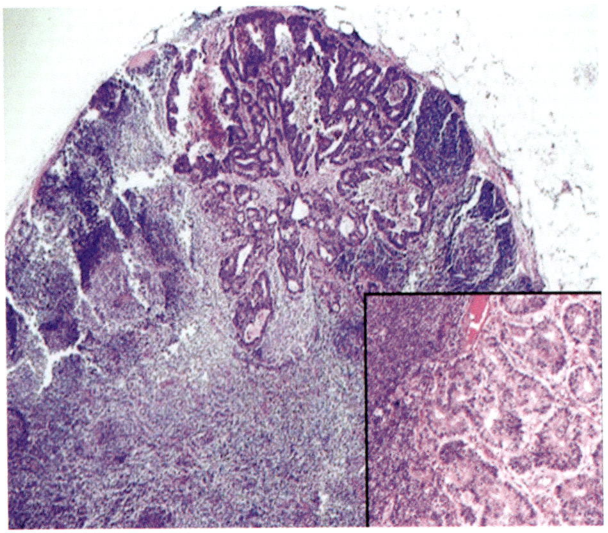

Figure 19: Metastatic adenocarcinoma lymph node—Photomicrograph displaying a lymph node with partial effacement of architecture replaced by tumor glands. Inset showing higher magnification of tumor glands.

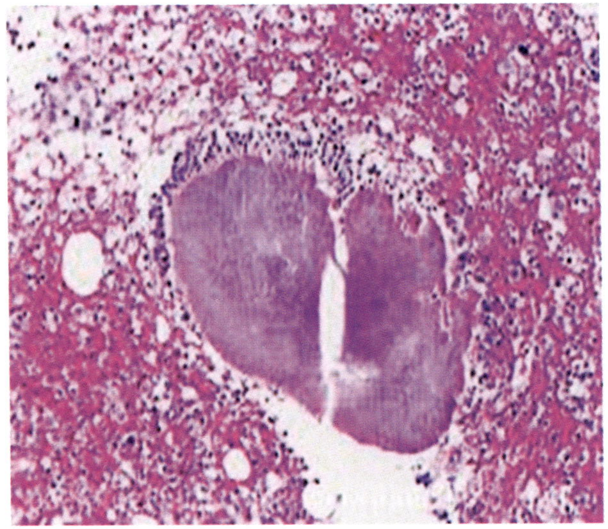

Figure 20: Actinomycosis—Photomicrograph displaying microcolony of *Actinomyces sp.* surrounded by neutrophilic infiltrate.

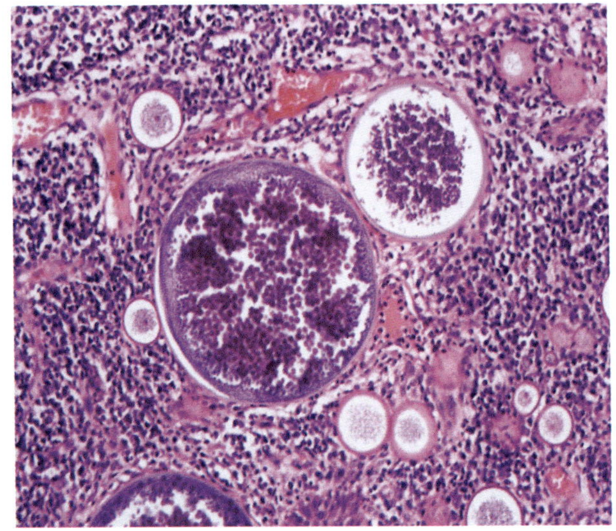

Figure 21: Rhinosporidiosis—Photomicrograph displaying multiple sporangia of *Rhinosporidium seeberi* embedded in stroma with dense inflammation.

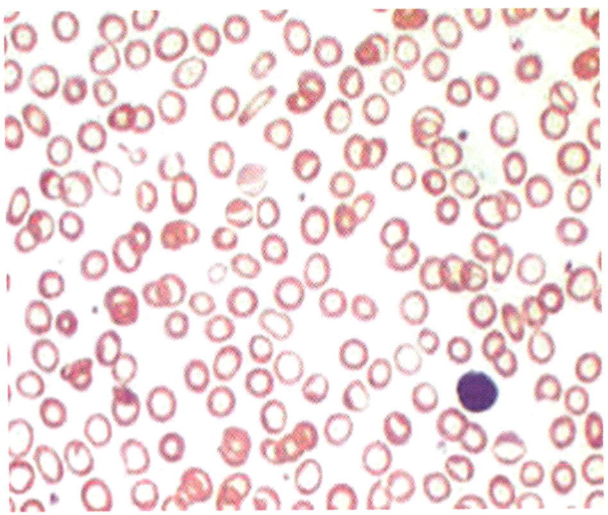

Figure 22: Iron deficiency anemia—Photomicrograph displaying microcytic and hypochromic with occasional pencil shaped erythrocytes. A small lymphocyte is also seen for comparison with size of erythrocytes.

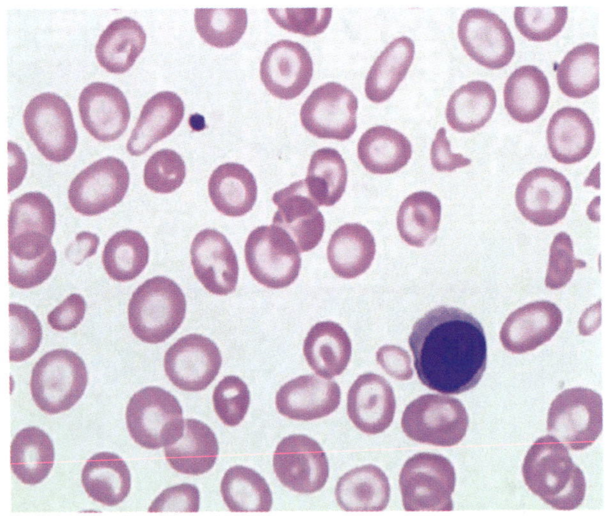

Figure 23: Thalassemia—Photomicrograph displaying microcytic hypochromic erythrocytes with many target cells.

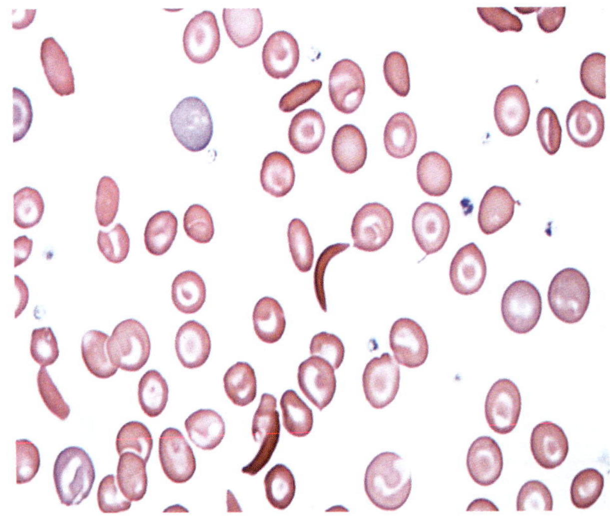

Figure 24: Sickle cell anemia—Photomicrograph displaying sickle shaped erythrocytes with target cells.

Plate 5

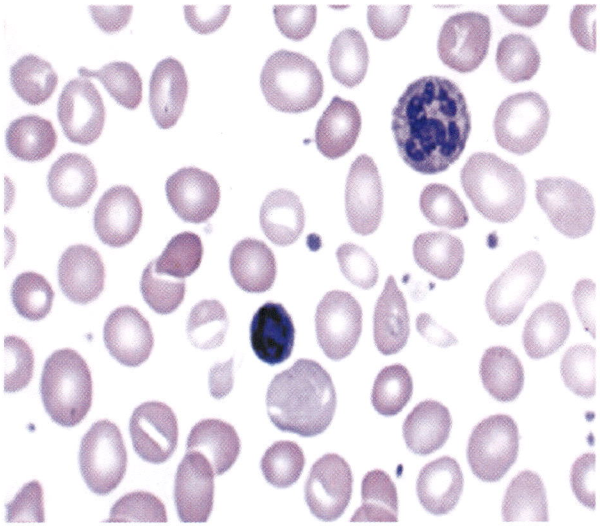

Figure 25: Macrocytic anemia—Photomicrograph displaying macroovalocytic erythrocytes, teardrop cells and hypersegmented neutrophils.

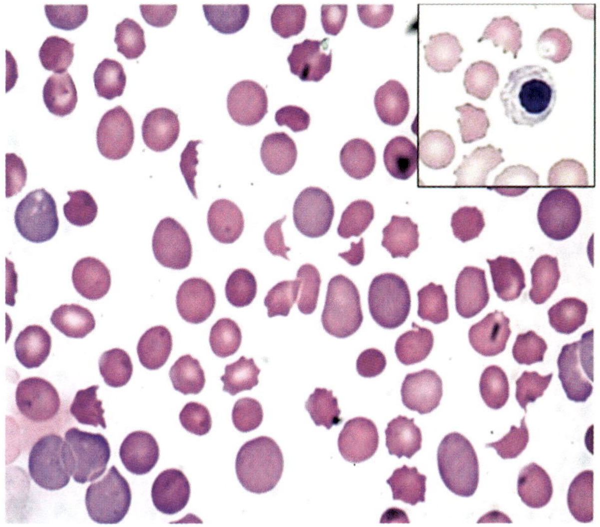

Figure 26: Hemolytic anemia—Photomicrograph displaying fragmented erythrocytes (schistocytes), polychromatophilic RBCs and nucleated RBCs (Inset).

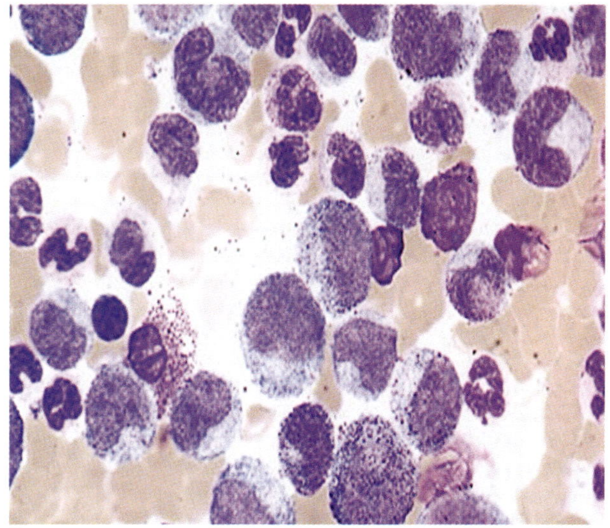

Figure 27: Chronic myeloid leukemia—Photomicrograph displaying high total leucocyte count with shift to left of myeloid series of cells comprising promyelocytes, myelocytes, metamyelocytes and band forms associated with eosinophilia.

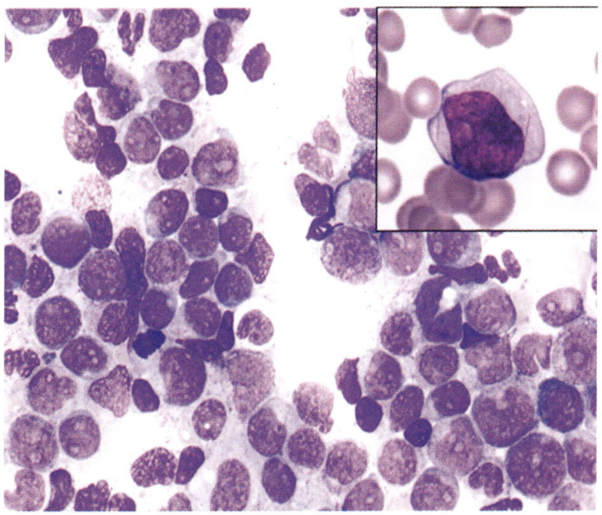

Figure 28: Acute myeloid leukemia—Photomicrograph displaying increased total leucocyte count with two Auer rods predominance of seen in cytoplasm of myeloblast (Inset).

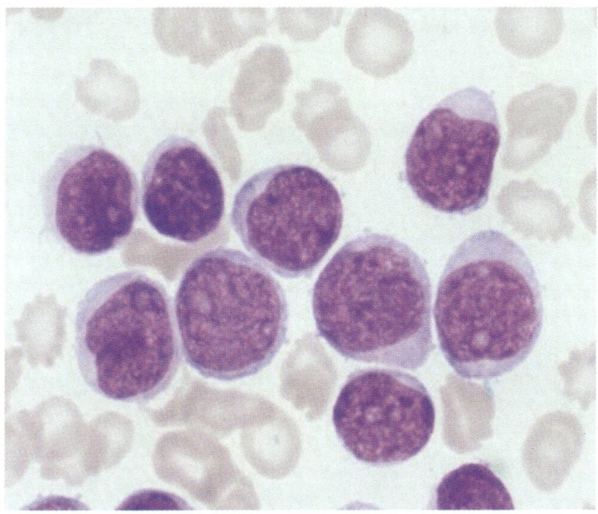

Figure 29: Acute lymphoblastic leukemia—Photomicrograph displaying increased total leucocyte count with predominance of lymphoblasts.

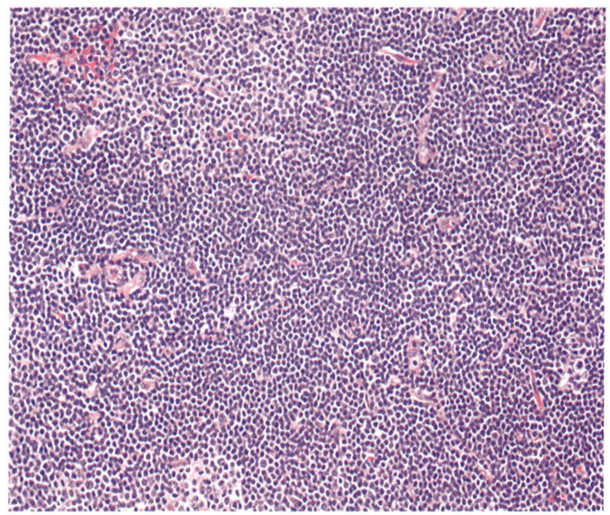

Figure 30: Non-Hodgkin lymphoma—Photomicrograph effacement of lymph node architecture with monotonous myeloblasts. Sheets of small lymphoid cells.

Plate 6

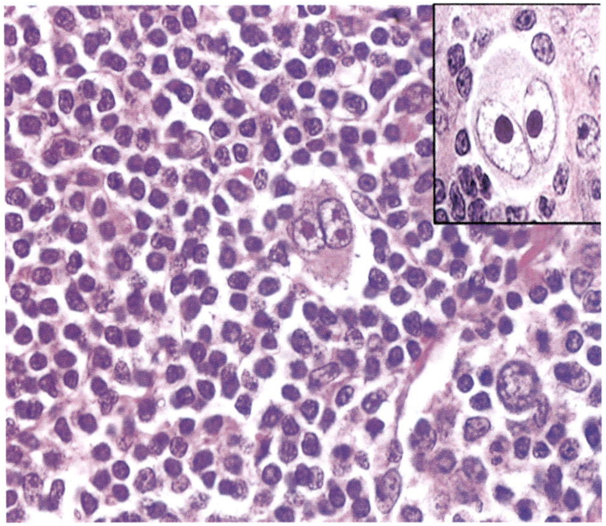

Figure 31: Hodgkin lymphoma—Photomicrograph displaying binucleate Reed-Sternberg cell (Higher magnification in inset), mononuclear Hodgkin cell and sheets of lymphocytes.

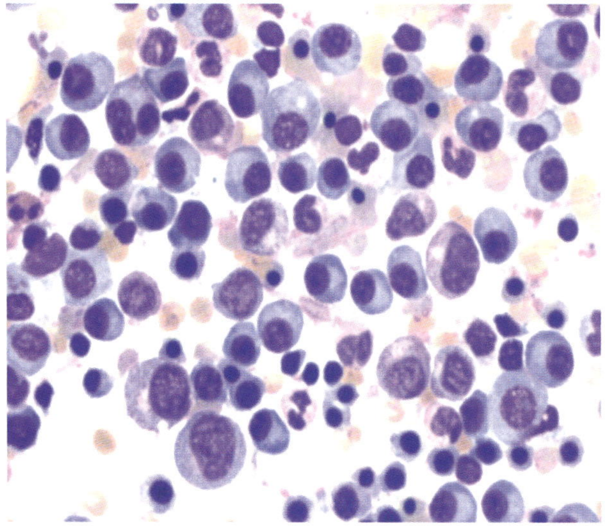

Figure 32: Multiple myeloma—Photomicrograph of bone marrow displaying sheets of plasma (Myeloma) cells.

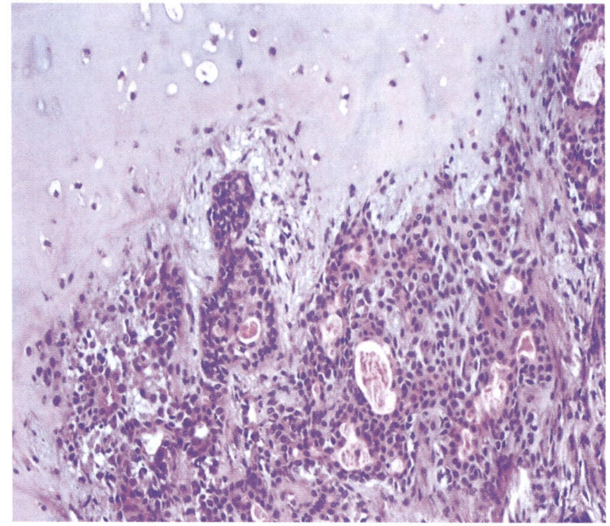

Figure 33: Pleomorphic adenoma—Photomicrograph displaying admixture of epithelial cells in ductular pattern, spindle shaped myoepithelial cells and chondromyxoid stroma (above).

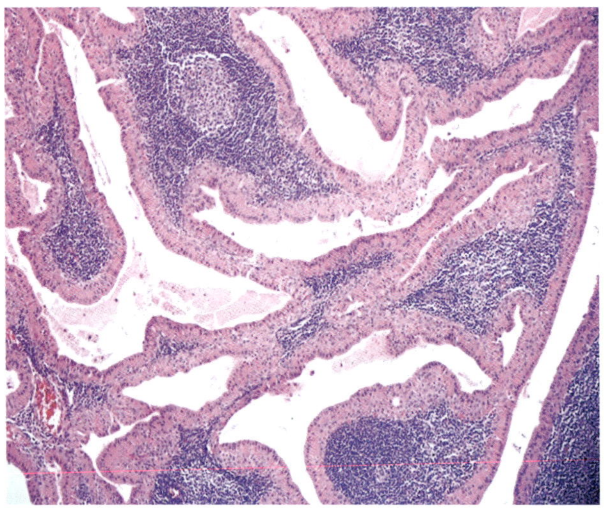

Figure 34: Warthin tumor—Photomicrograph displaying papillary fronds lined by double cell layered tall columnar epithelium with dense lymphocytic infiltration in stroma and formation of germinal centres.

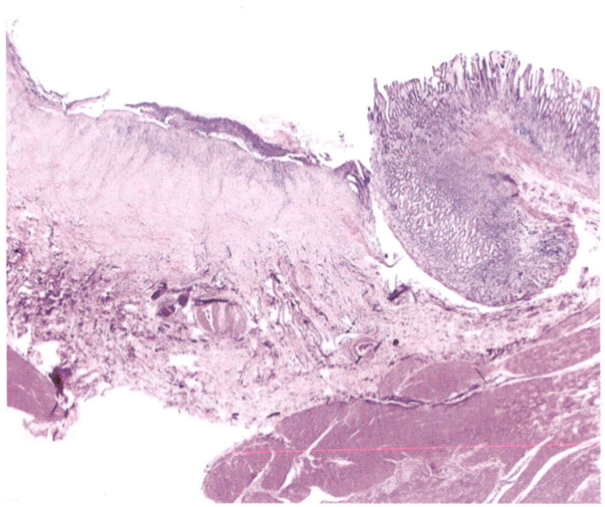

Figure 35: Peptic ulcer—Photomicrograph displaying edge of ulcer with luminal purulent exudate, fibrinoid necrosis, granulation tissue formation and fibrosis (in muscularis) from top to bottom.

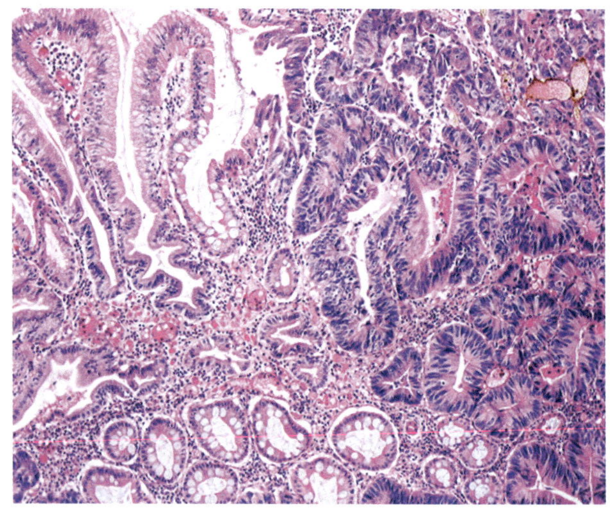

Figure 36: Gastric adenocarcinoma—Photomicrograph displaying normal gastric mucosa (Left) with tumor cells arranged in glands (Right).

Plate 7

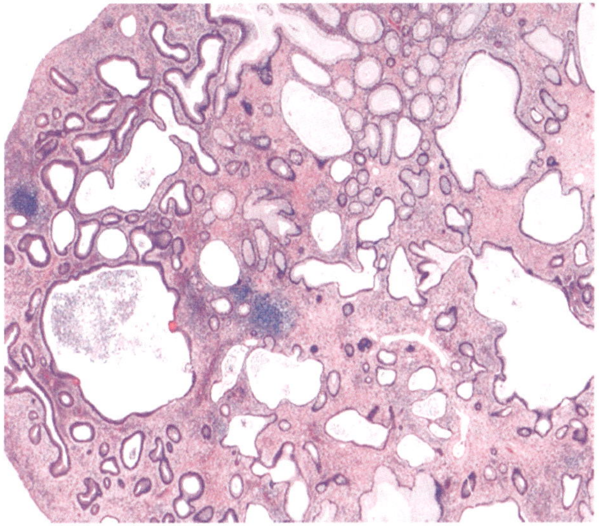

Figure 37: Juvenile rectal polyp—Photomicrograph displaying cystically dilated glands lined by tall columnar epithelium with intervening fibrous stroma.

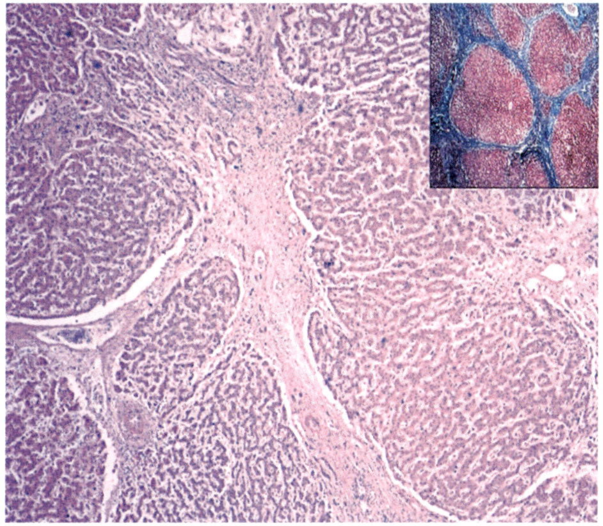

Figure 38: Cirrhosis—Photomicrograph displaying regenerating hepatocytic nodules separated by dense fibrous septae. Masson trichrome stain displaying prominent fibrosis (blue in inset).

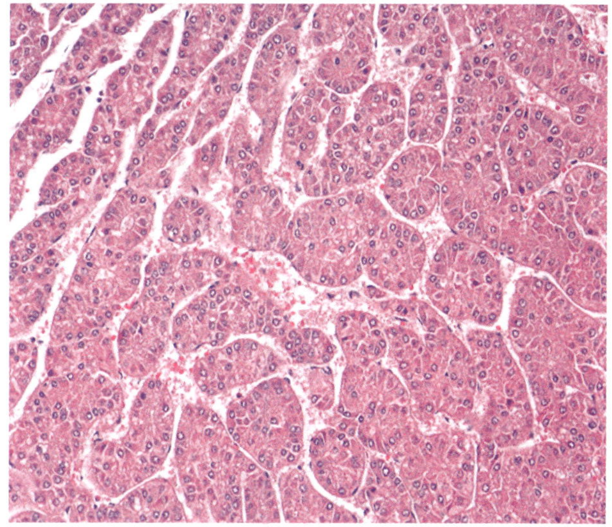

Figure 38: Hepatocellular carcinoma—Photomicrograph displaying nests and trabeculae of malignant hepatocytic tumor cells.

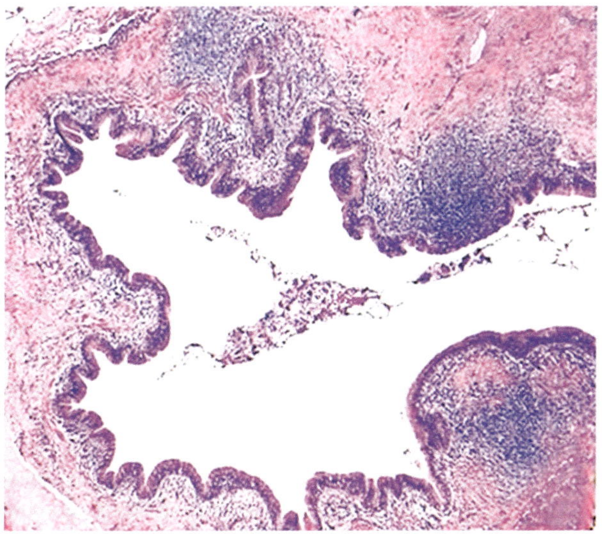

Figure 40: Bronchiectasis—Photomicrograph displaying dilated bronchiole with lymphoid follicles in subepithelial stroma.

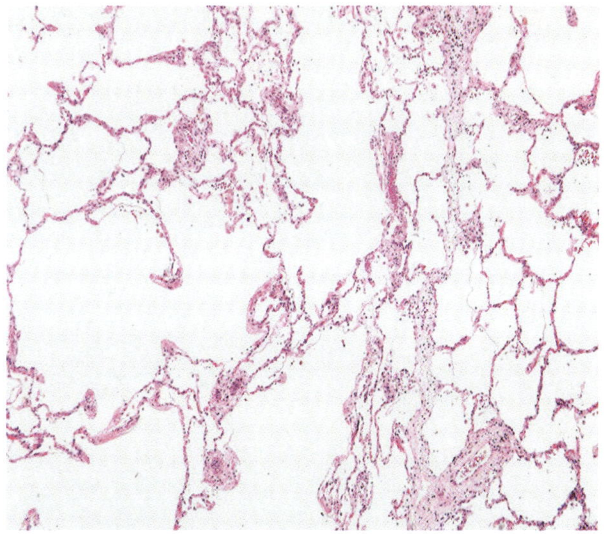

Figure 41: Emphysema—Photomicrograph displaying variably dilated alveolar sacs with destruction of their walls and interstitial inflammation.

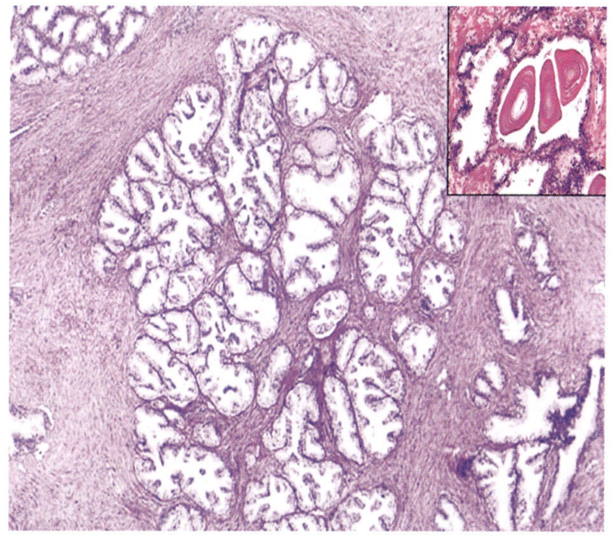

Figure 42: Benign prostatic hypertrophy—Photomicrograph displaying fibromuscular hypertrophy and glandular hyperplasia. Corpora amylacea seen in lumen of glands (Inset).

Plate 8

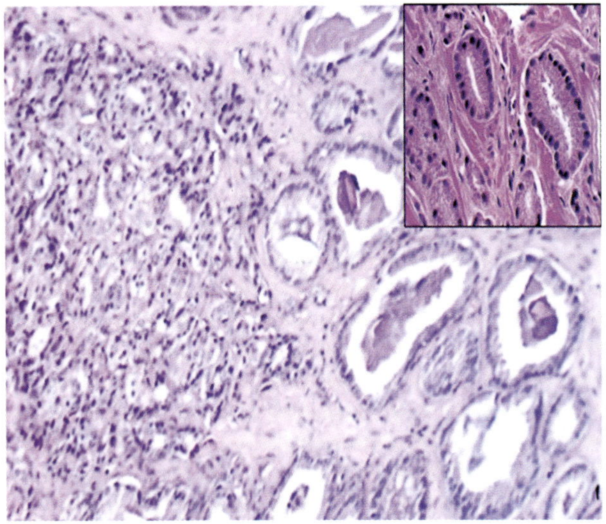

Figure 43: Carcinoma prostate—Photomicrograph displaying tumor cells in microglandular pattern and nests (Left). Tumor glands are lined by single layer of cells and lack myoepithelial cell layer (Inset).

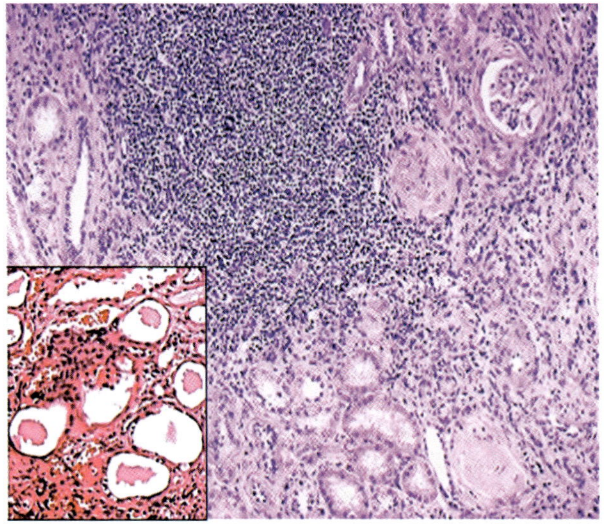

Figure 44: Chronic pyelonephritis—Photomicrograph displaying sclerosed glomeruli, tubular atrophy and interstial lymphocytic infiltrate. Thyroidisation of tubules seen in inset.

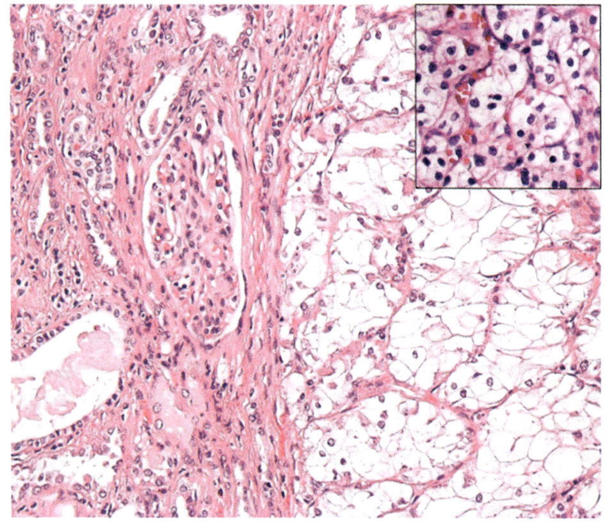

Figure 45: Renal cell carcinoma— Photomicrograph displaying a malignant tumor composed of clear cells (Right) with normal renal tissue (left). Higher magnification of clear tumor cells (inset).

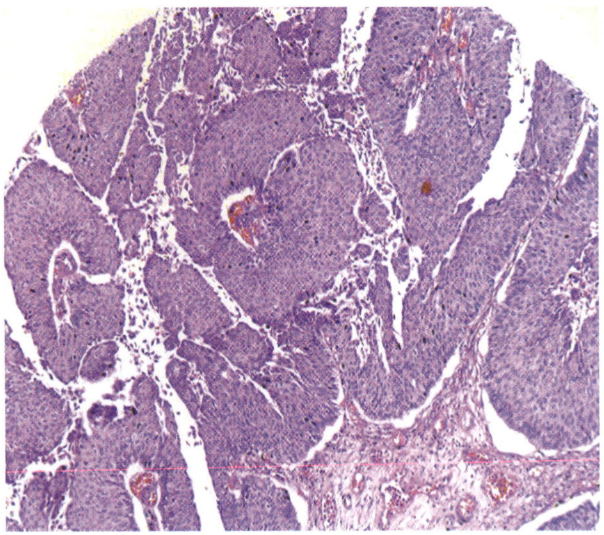

Figure 46: Urothelial carcinoma—Photomicrograph displaying papillary fronds lined by highly pleomorphic urothelial tumor cells.

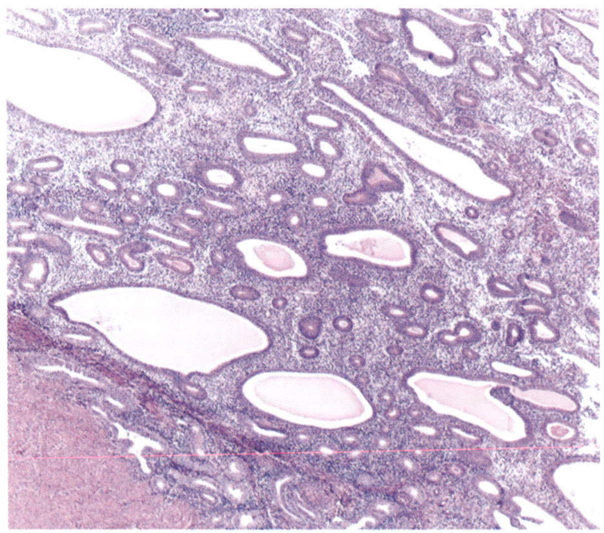

Figure 47: Simple endometrial hyperplasia—Photomicrograph displaying small to cystically dilated hyperplastic endometrial glands.

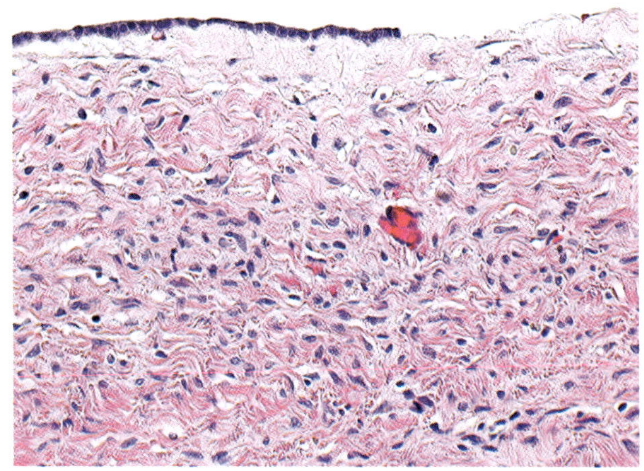

Figure 48: Serous cystadenoma—Photomicrograph displaying a fibrocollagenous cyst wall lined by ciliated low columnar epithelium.

Plate 9

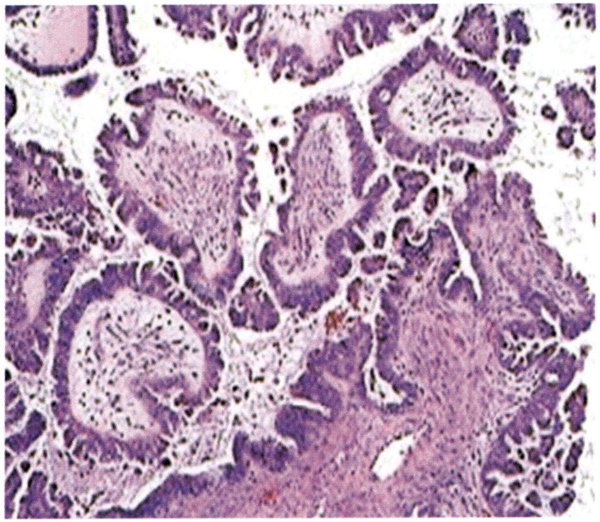

Figure 49: Papillary serous cystadenocarcinoma—Photomicrograph displaying papillary fronds lined by tumor cells with invasion into the subepithelial stroma.

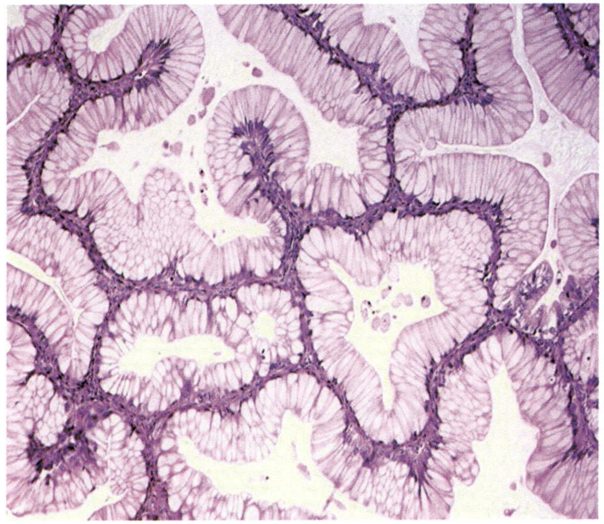

Figure 50: Mucinous cystadenoma—Photomicrograph displaying large cystically dilated glands lined by mucin secreting nonciliated tall columnar epithelium.

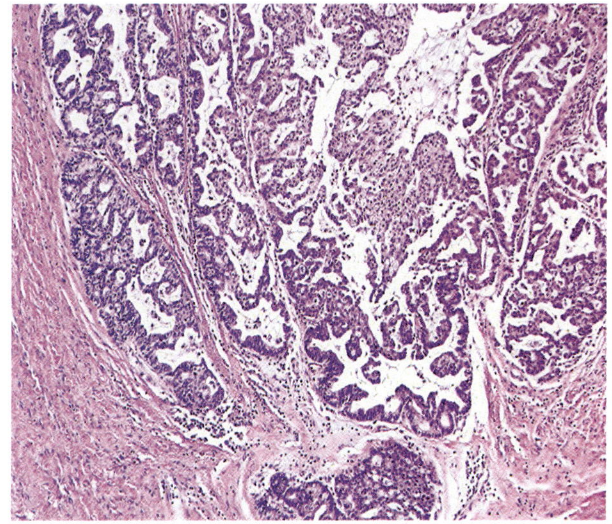

Figure 51: Mucinous cystadenocarcinoma—Photomicrograph displaying solid and cystic areas lined by pleomorphic tumor cells with stromal invasion.

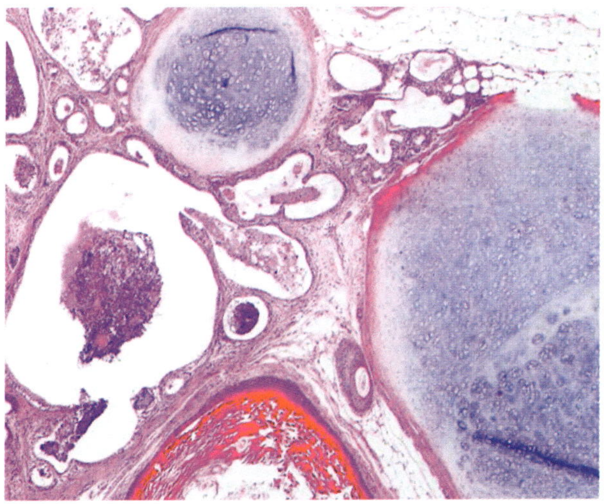

Figure 52: Mature cystic teratoma—Photomicrograph displaying helter skelter collection of mature hyaline cartilage, keratinous cyst line by stratified squamous epithelium, sebaceous glands with hair follicle and adipose tissue.

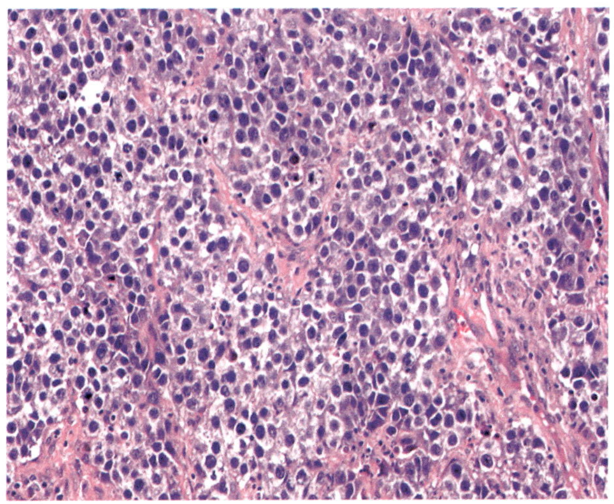

Figure 53: Dysgerminoma—Photomicrograph displaying sheets of polygonal cells with monomorphic nuclei and pale cytoplasm separated by fibrous septae containing lymphocytes.

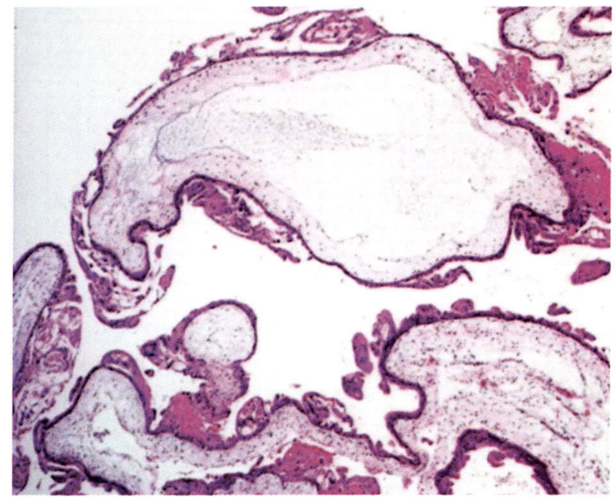

Figure 54: Hydatidiform mole—Photomicrograph displaying chorionic villi with hydropic degeneration, avascularity, cistern formation and circumferential trophoblastic proliferation.

Plate 10

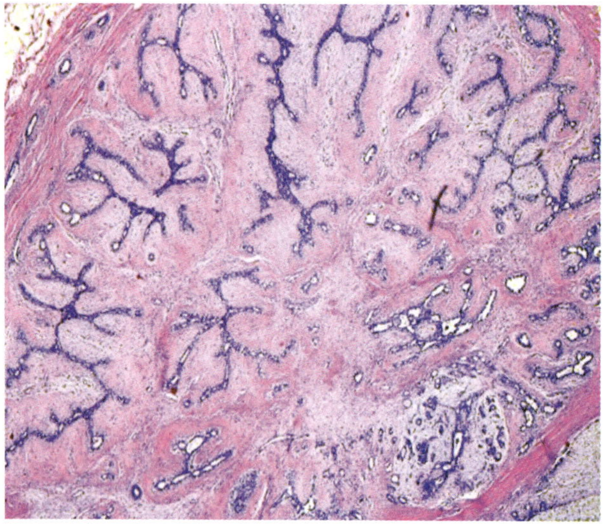

Figure 55: Fibroadenoma—Photomicrograph displaying encapsulation, proliferation of fibrous stroma with myxoid areas, compressed elongated ducts and tubular ducts lined by double layered epithelium.

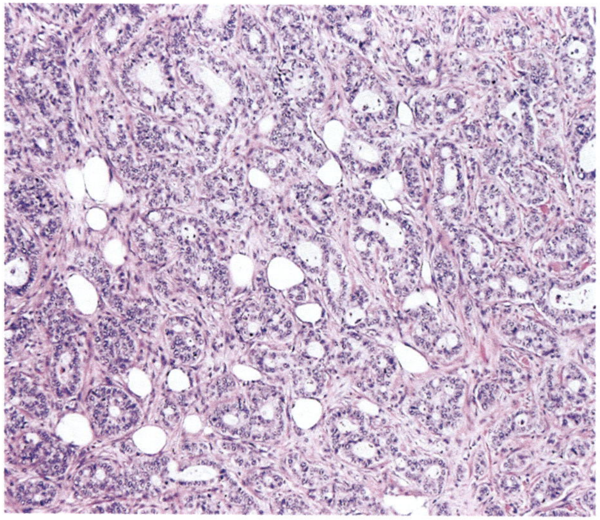

Figure 56: Invasive ductal carcinoma breast—Photomicrograph displaying tubules and nests of pleomorphic tumor cells. Within the ducts, myoepithelial cells are absent.

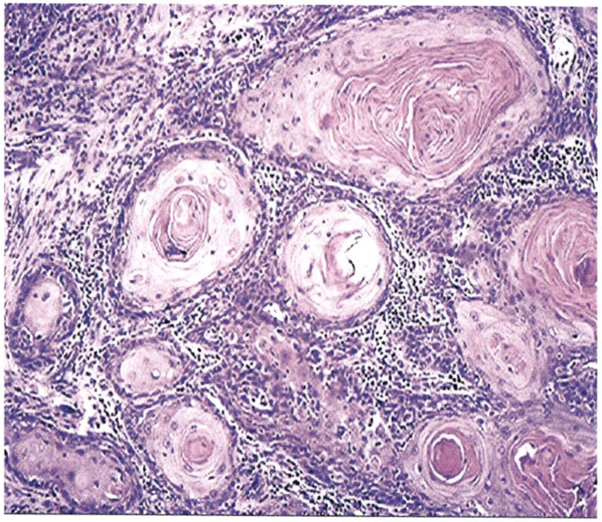

Figure 57: Squamous cell carcinoma—Photomicrograph displaying nests of pleomorphic tumor cells with keratin pearls in between.

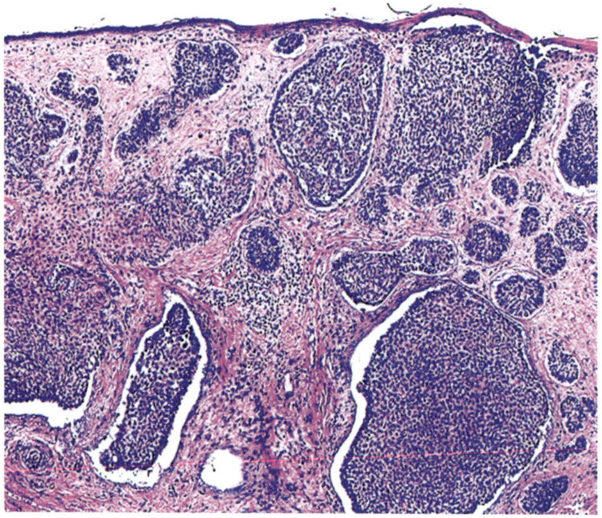

Figure 58: Basal cell carcinoma—Photomicrograph displaying nests of basophilic tumor cells with peripheral palisading and separation clefts from surrounding stroma. Epidermis is atrophic.

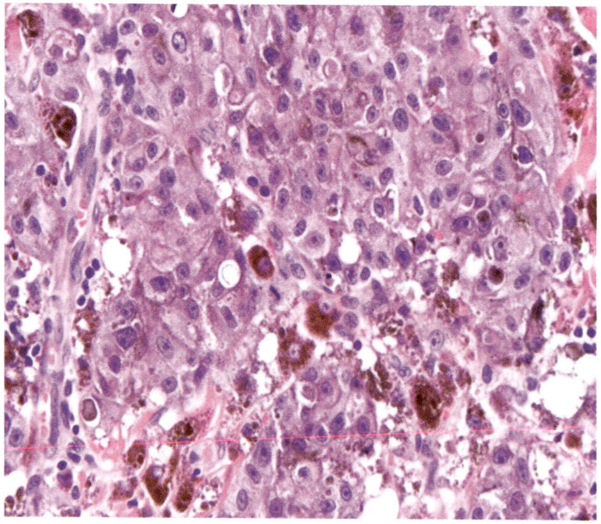

Figure 58: Malignant melanoma—Photomicrograph displaying nests and sheets of tumor cells with prominent eosinophilic nucleoli. Variable amount of melanin seen.

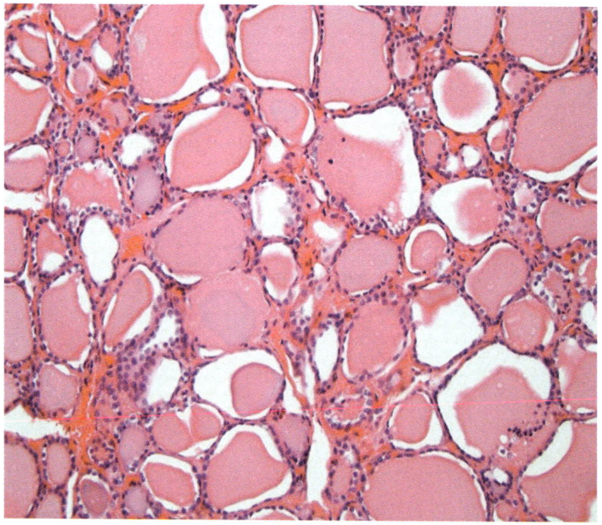

Figure 60: Nodular colloid goitre—Photomicrograph displaying variable sized follicles lined by flattened follicular epithelial cells with luminal eosinophilic colloid.

Plate 11

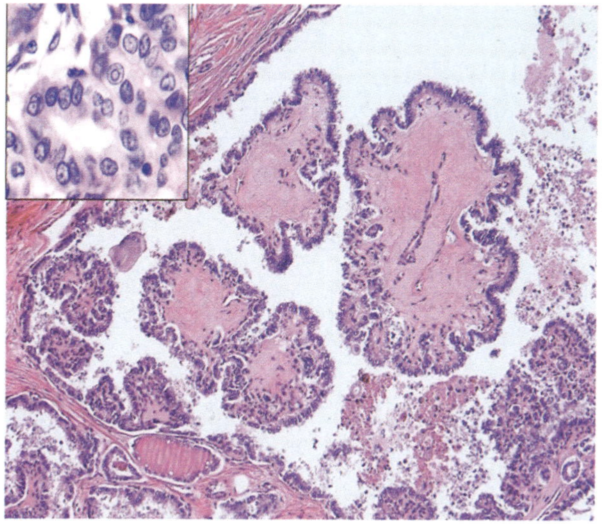

Figure 61: Papillary carcinoma of thyroid—Photomicrograph displaying papillae lined by neoplastic cell displaying nuclear crowding and overlapping. Individual tumor cells show ground glass nuclei with grooving and pseudonucleoli (Inset).

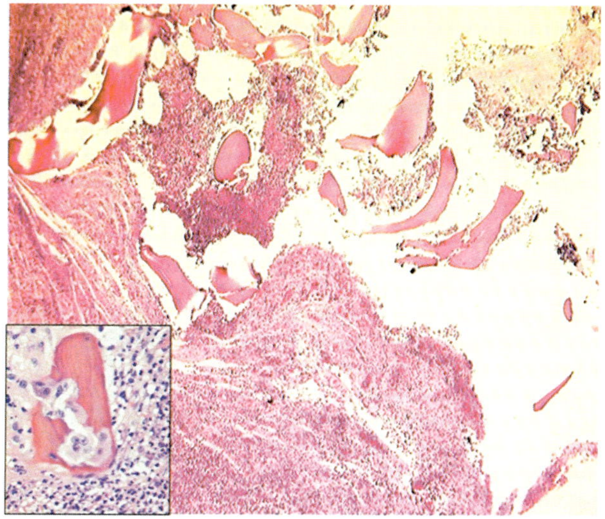

Figure 62: Pyogenic osteomyelitis—Photomicrograph displaying sequestrum (Inset), involucrum and dense neutrophilic infiltrate in surrounding stroma.

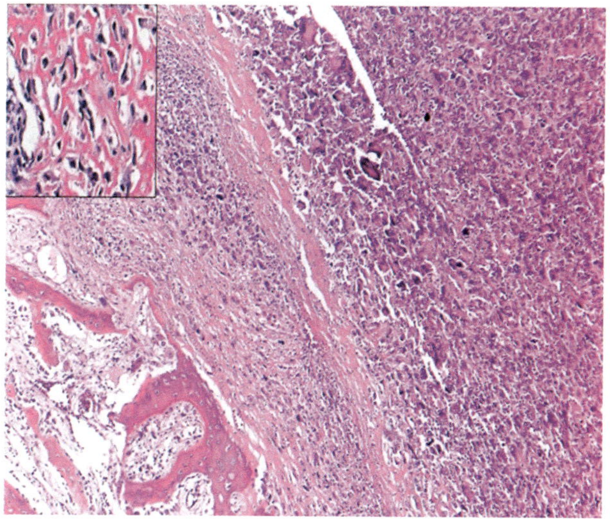

Figure 63: Osteosarcoma—Photomicrograph displaying pleomorphic tumor cells with malignant osteoid (Right) with normal bony trabeculae (Left). Coarse lace like malignant osteoid seen in inset.

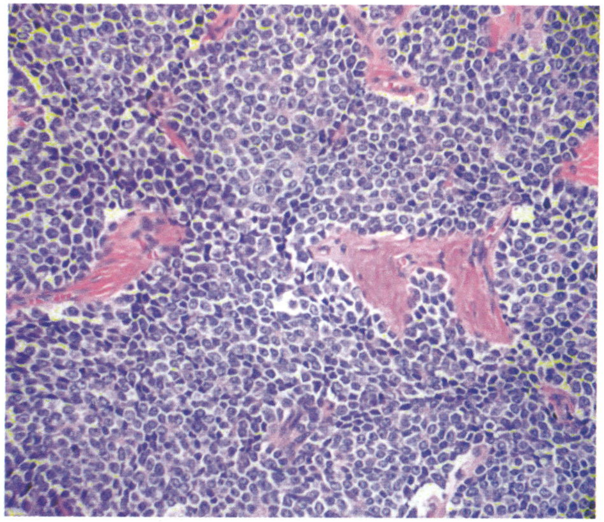

Figure 64: Ewing sarcoma—Photomicrograph displaying small round neoplastic cells having scanty cytoplasm in sheets separated by fibrous bands.

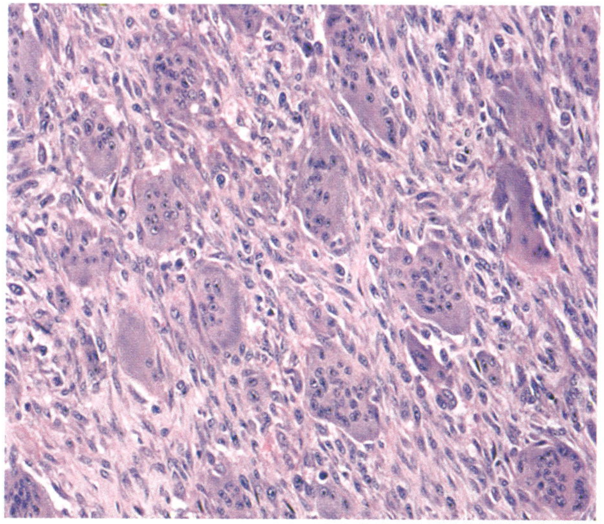

Figure 65: Osteoclastoma—Photomicrograph displaying syncytial sheets of uniform oval mononuclear cells with numerous osteoclast-like giant cells.

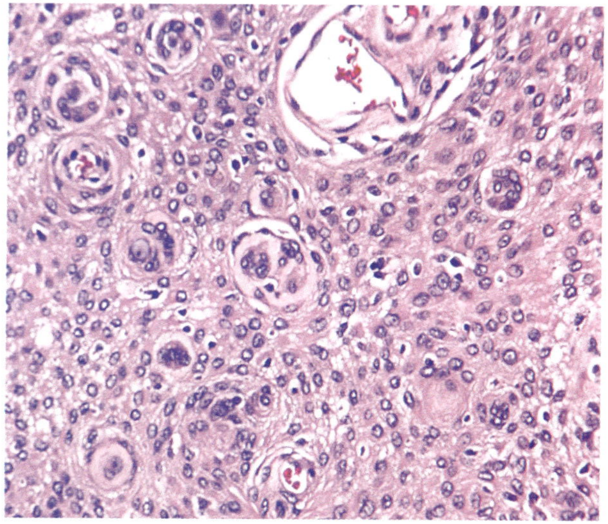

Figure 66: Meningioma—Photomicrograph displaying sheets of meningothelial cells having high N:C ratio with formation of many meningothelial whorls.

Plate 12

Gross Pathology

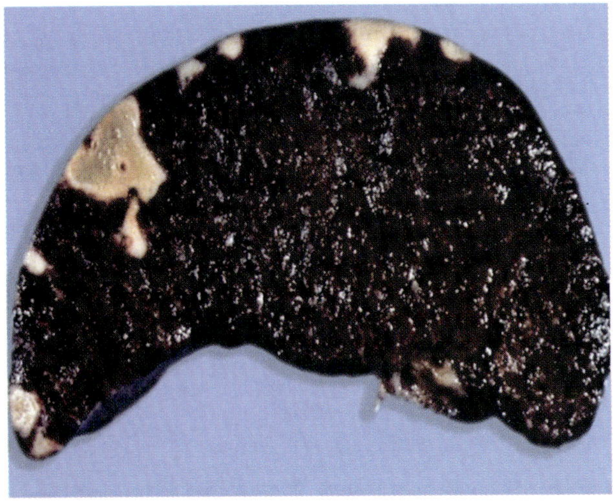

Image A: Coagulative necrosis

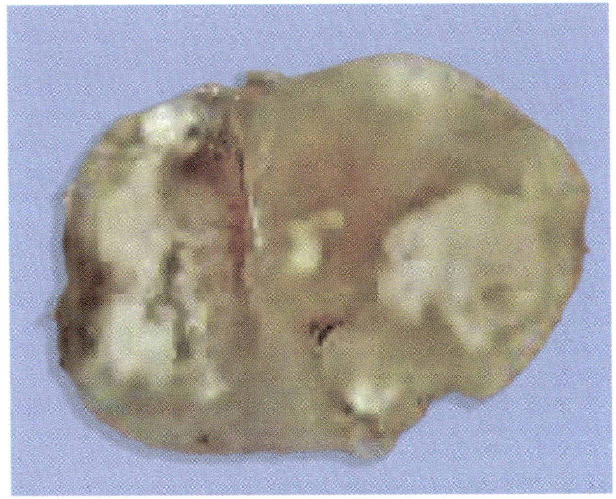

Image B: Caseous necrosis

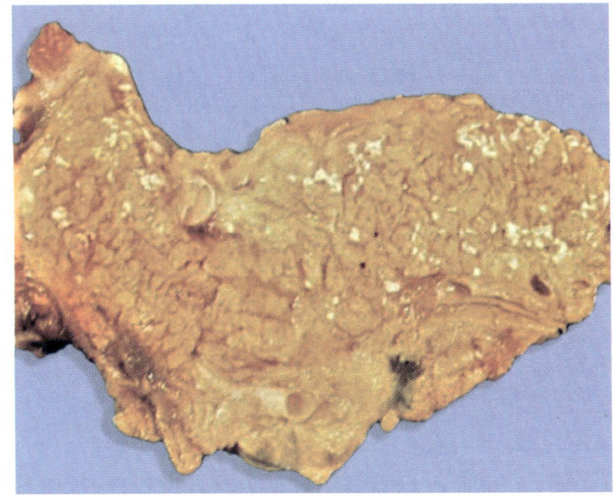

Image C: Fat necrosis

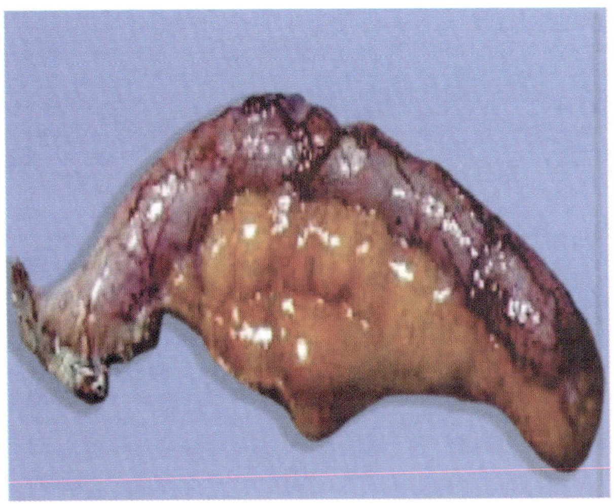

Image D: Acute appendicitis

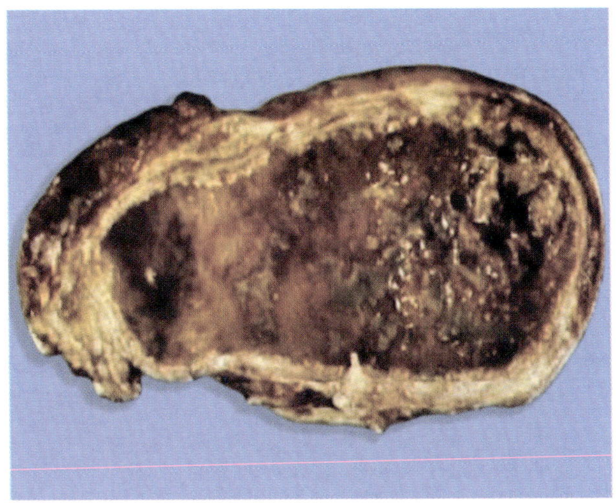

Image E: Chronic cholecystitis

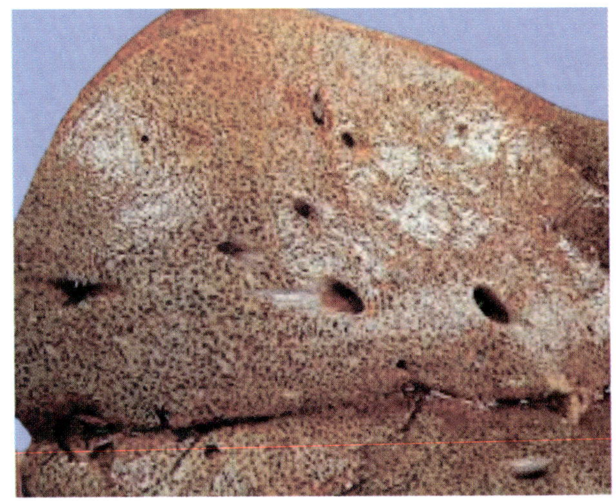

Image F: Chronic venous congestion liver

Plate 13

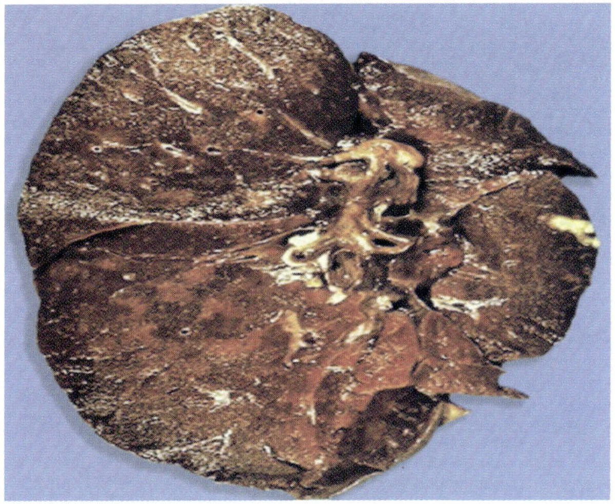

Image G: Primary pulmonary tuberculosis

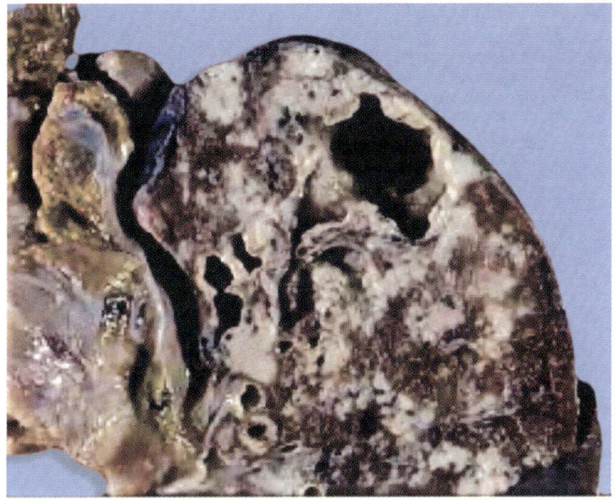

Image H: Secondary pulmonary tuberculosis

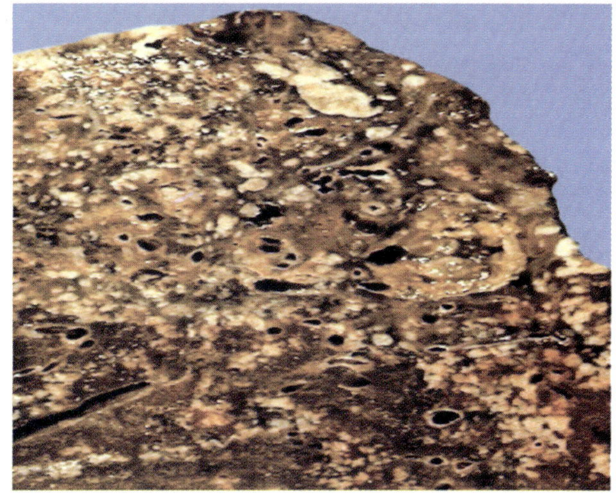

Image I: Miliary tuberculosis

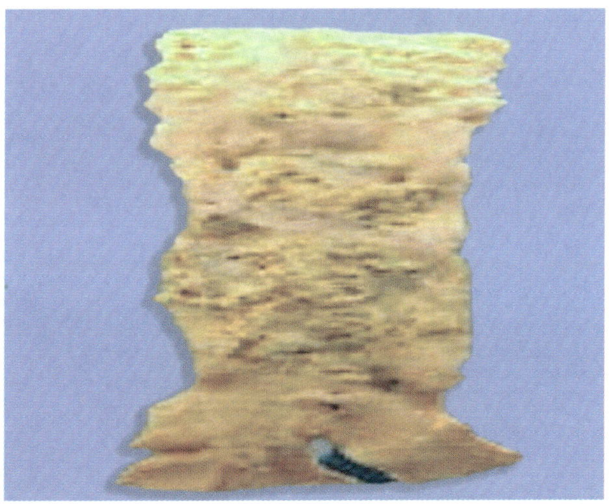

Image J: Atherosclerosis aorta

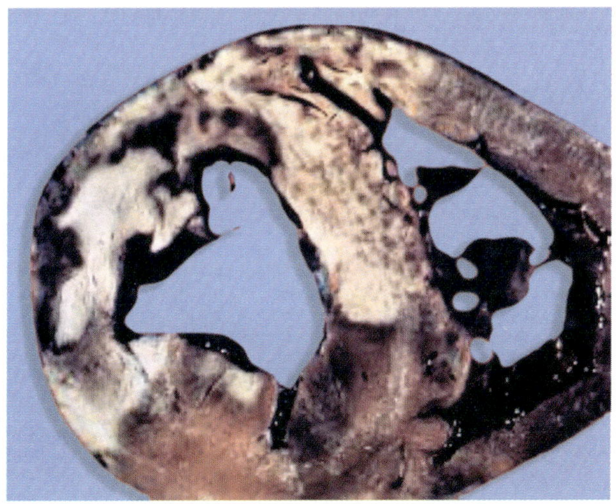

Image K: Myocardial infarction

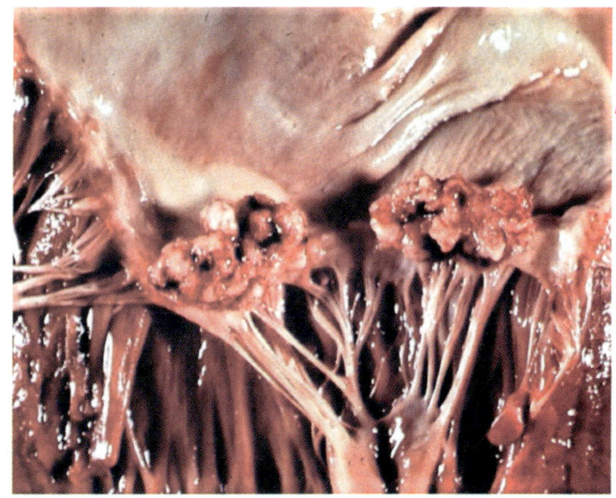

Image L: Vegetations in infective endocarditis

Plate 14

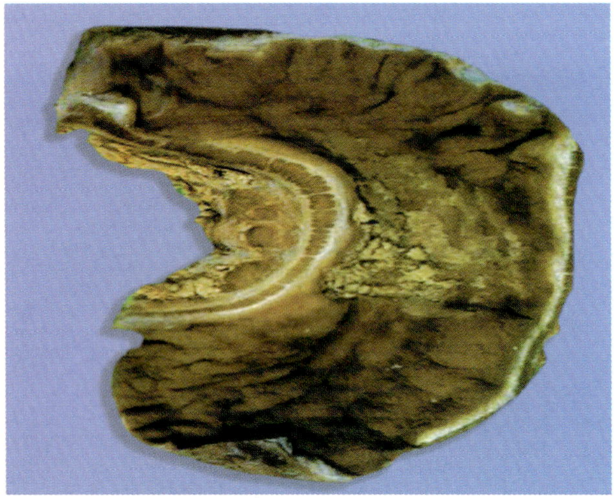

Image M: Gastric carcinoma

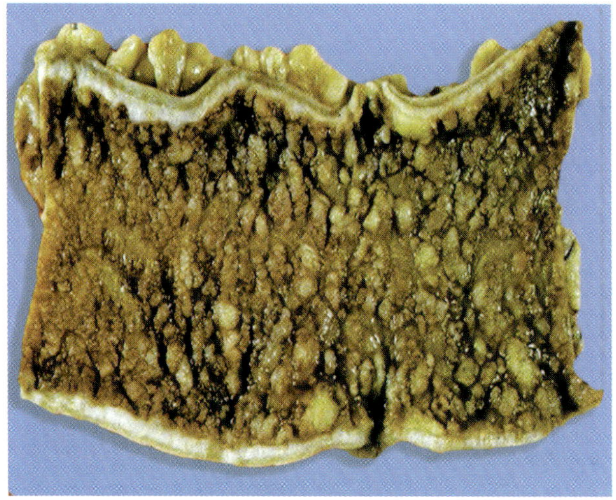

Image N: Crohn's disease

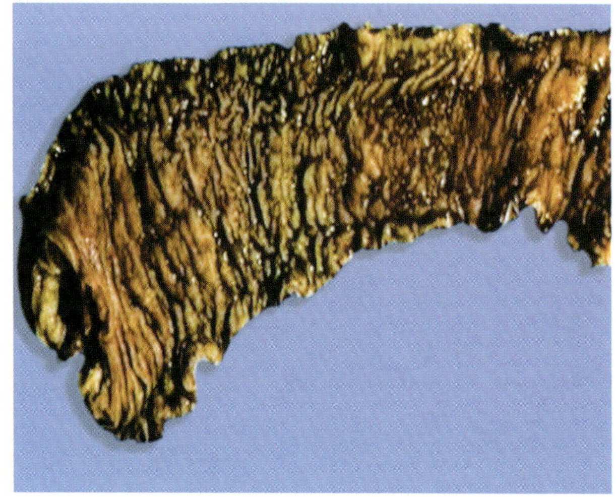

Image O: Ulcerative colitis

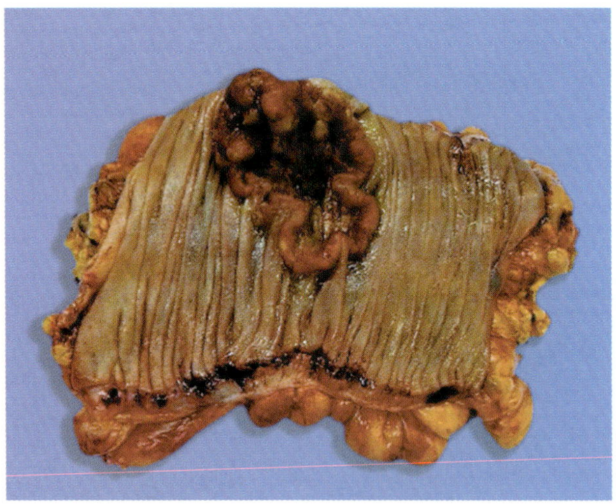

Image P: Colorectal carcinoma

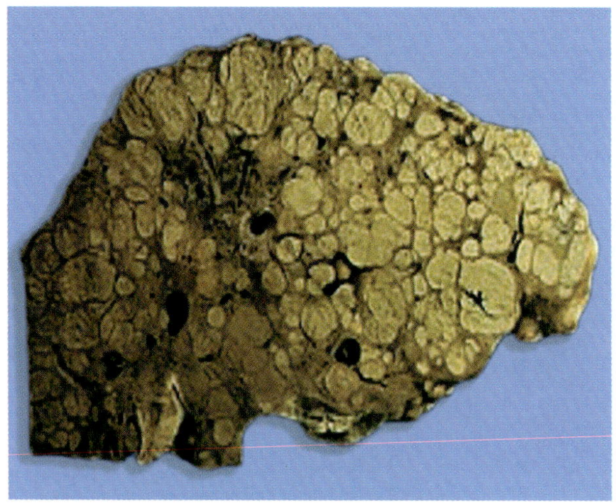

Image Q: Hepatic cirrhosis

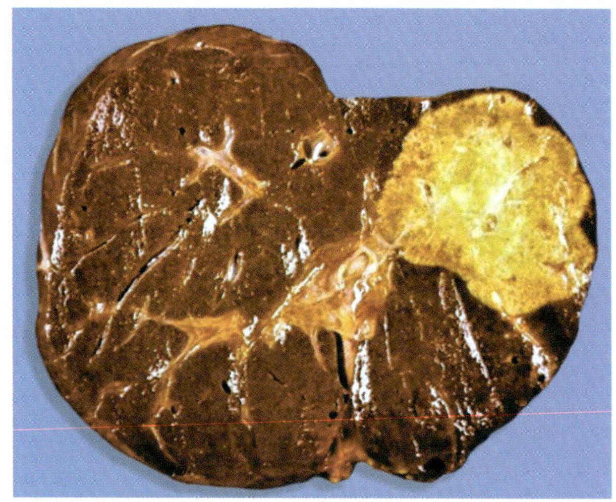

Image R: Hepatocellular carcinoma

Plate 15

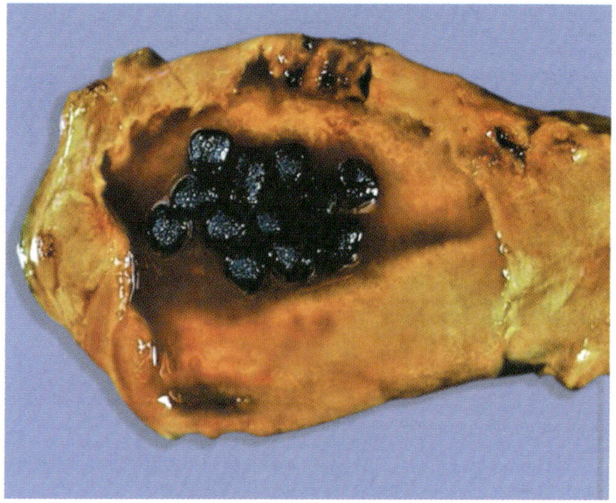

Image S: Cholelithiasis

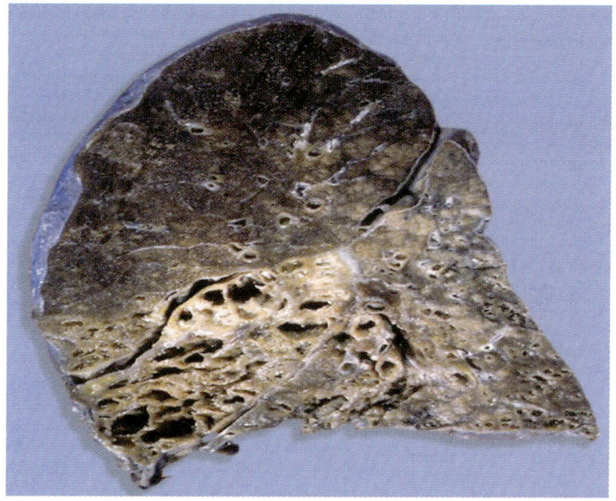

Image T: Bronchiectasis

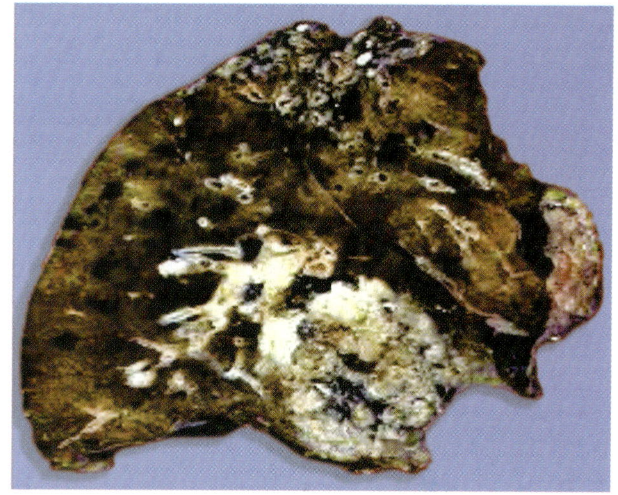

Image U: Bronchogenic carcinoma

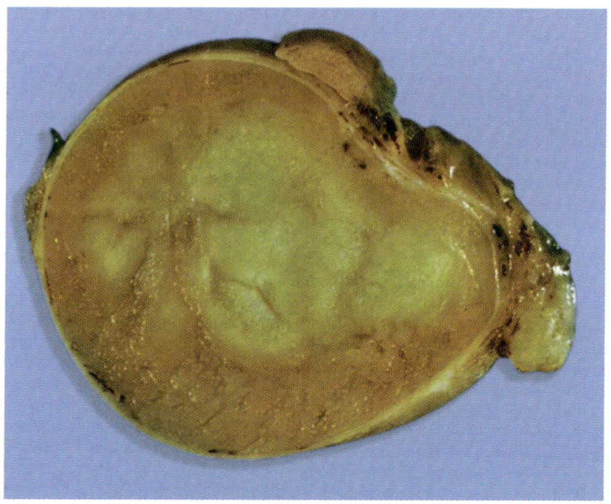

Image V: Seminoma testis

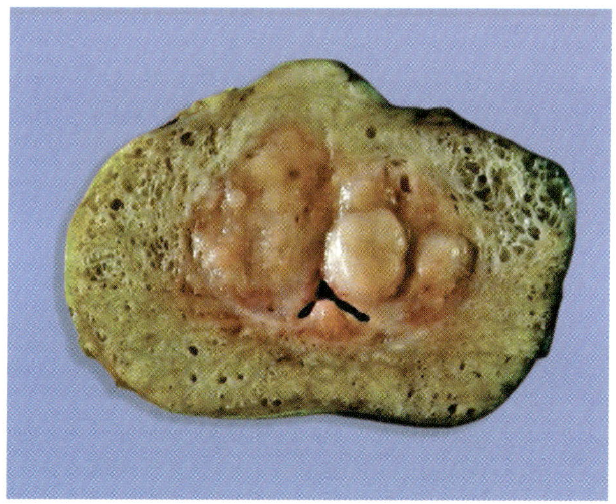

Image W: Benign prostatic hyperplasia

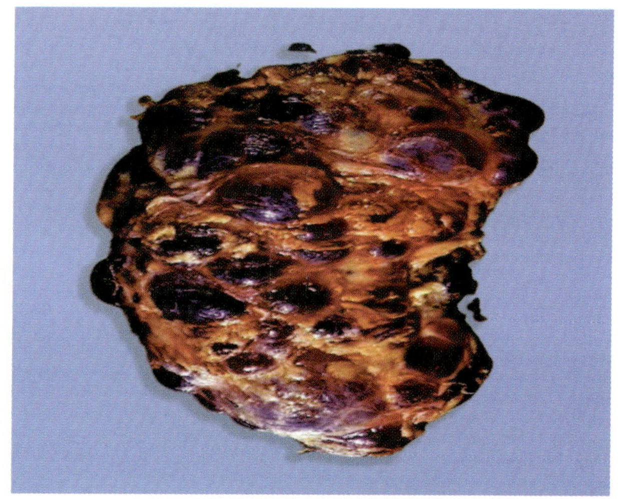

Image X: Adult polycystic kidney disease

Plate 16

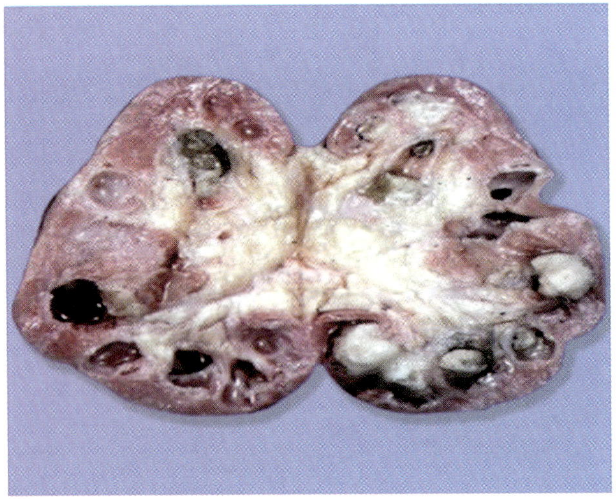
Image Y: Nephrolithiasis

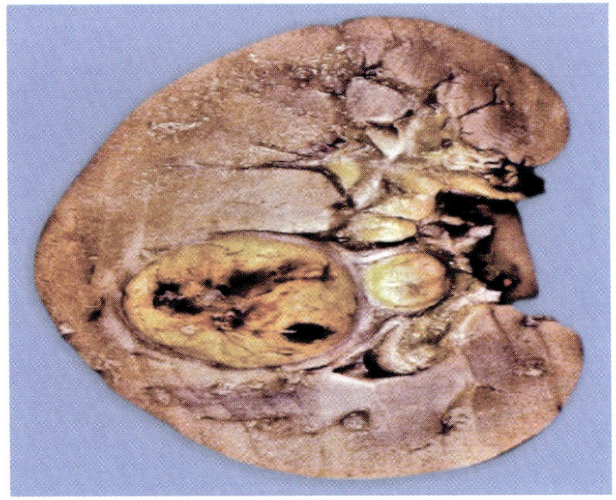
Image Z: Renal cell carcinoma

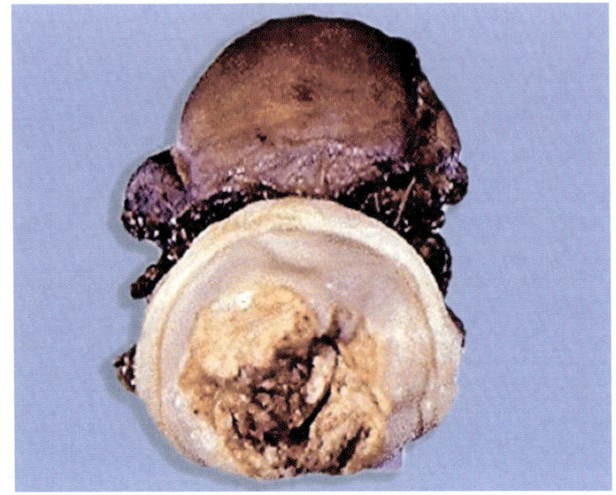
Image A1: Carcinoma cervix

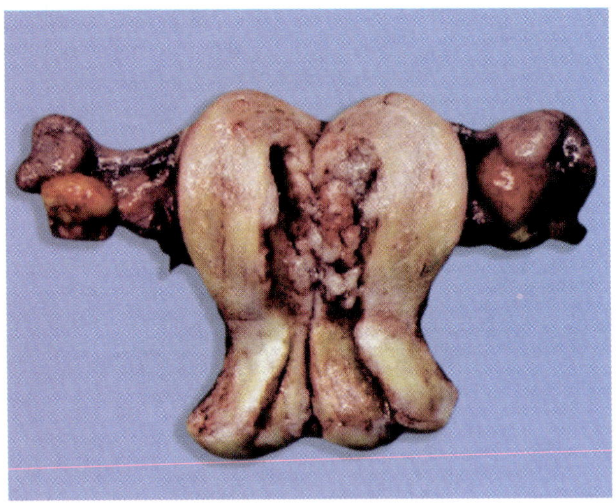
Image B1: Endometrial carcinoma

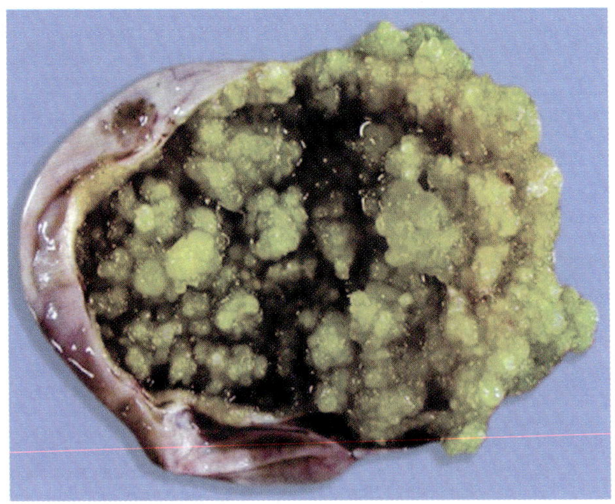
Image C1: Papillary serous cystadenocarcinoma

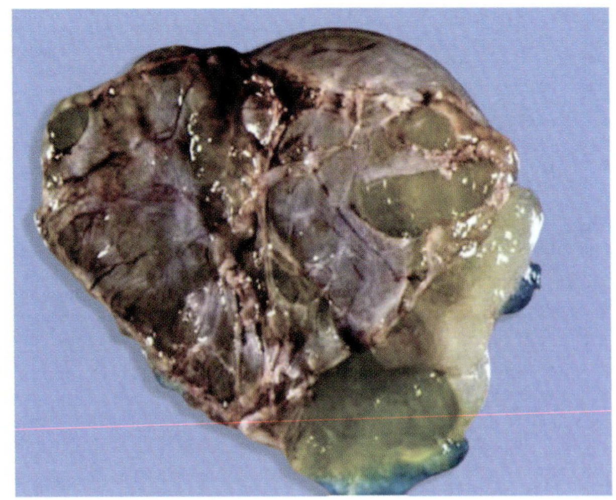
Image D1: Borderline mucinous neoplasm

Plate 17

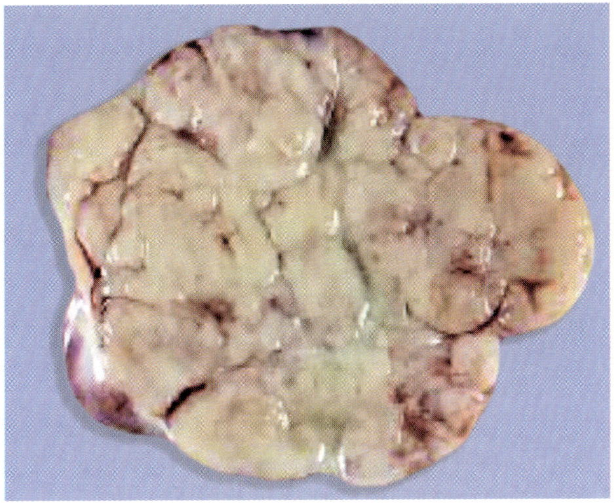

Image E1: Dysgerminoma

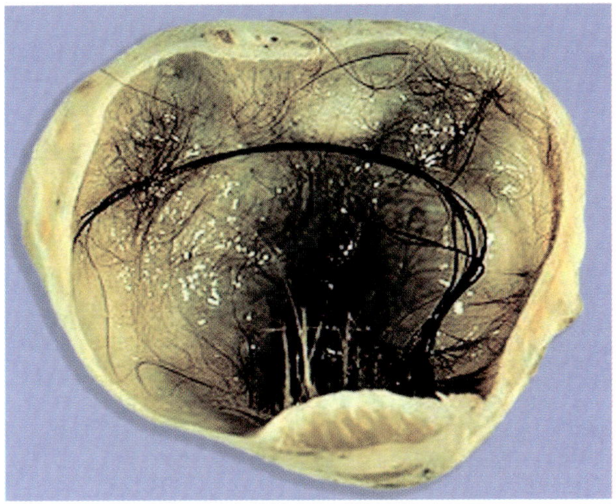

Image F1: Mature cystic teratoma

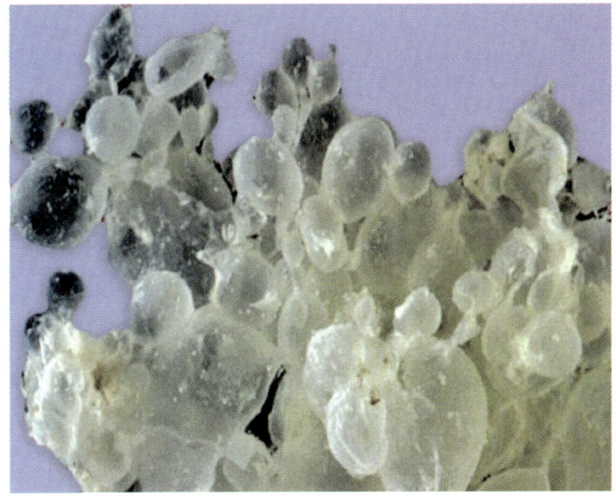

Image G1: Complete hydatidiform mole

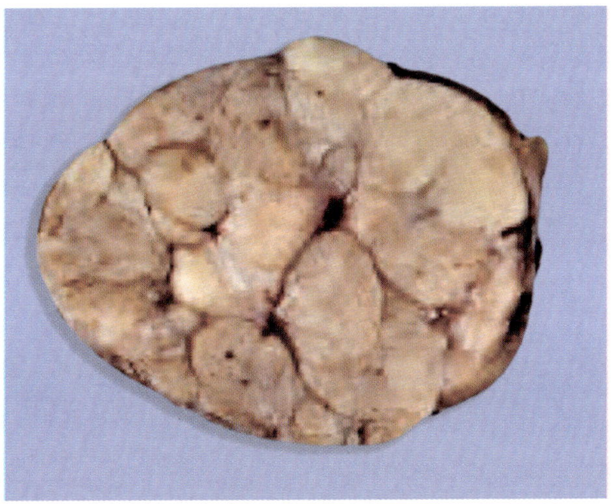

Image H1: Fibroadenoma

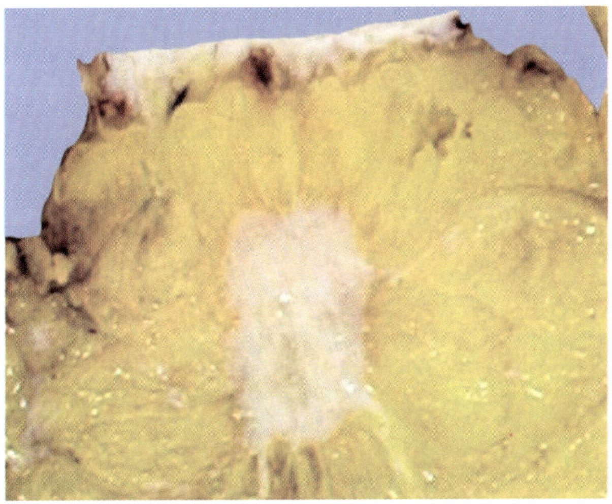

Image I1: Breast carcinoma

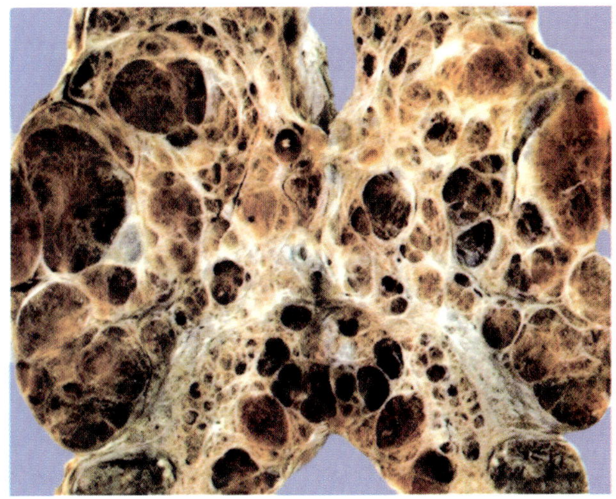

Image J1: Multinodular goitre

Plate 18

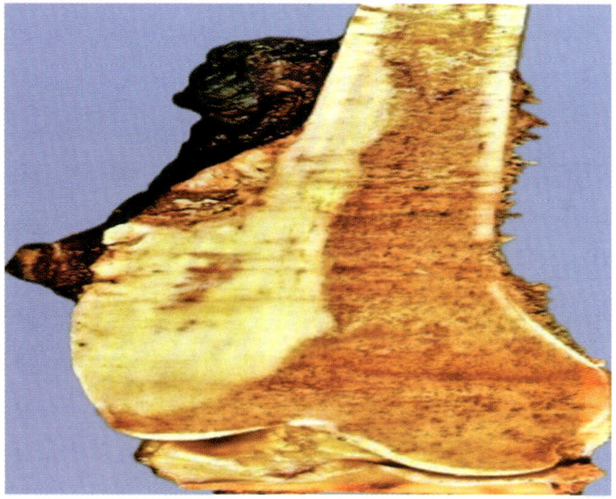

Image K1: Osteosarcoma

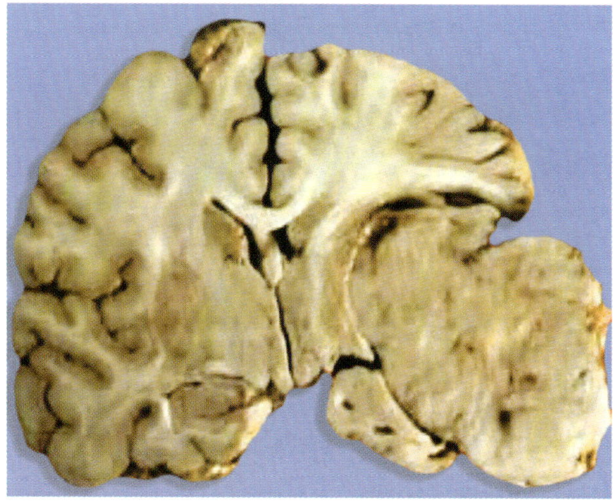

Image L1: Meningioma

CELLULAR EVENTS IN INFLAMMATION

Step I–Margination, rolling and adhesion of leucocytes to endothelium

Margination of leucocytes

- Due to stasis, leucocytes marginate to periphery of blood vessels
- Leucocytes tumble on endothelium, adhere and firmly attach to it.

Attachment of leucocytes to endothelium

- Attachment of leucocytes to endothelium occur by three families of adhesion molecules:
  - *Selectins*: They are a family of 3 closely related single chain glycoprotein, e.g. E-selectin is located on endothelium and binds with sialyl–Lewis X-receptor on neutrophils; P–selectin is located on endothelium and platelets and bind with sialyl–Lewis X-receptor on neutrophils; L–selectin is located on lymphocytes and bind with glycoprotein cell adhesion molecule-1 on endothelium
  - *Integrins*: They are a group of heterodimeric proteins composed of α and β chains located in leucocytes; β_2-integrin binds with intercellular adhesion molecule-1 on endothelium and β_1 integrins bind with vascular cell adhesion molecule-1 on endothelium
  - *Immunoglobulin super family*: It includes intercellular cell adhesion molecule-1, vascular cell adhesion molecule-1 and glycoprotein cell adhesion molecule-1 which bind with intergins on leucocytes.

Step II–Diapedesis (transmigration across endothelium)

- It occurs through interendothelial spaces under influence of chemokines
- CD31 located on endothelium helps in it
- Leucocytes pierce basement membrane with help of collagenases
- Leucocytes bind with extracellular matrix with help of integrins and CD44 on its surface.

Step III–Chemotaxis

- It is a process by which leucocytes travel towards focus of injury under chemical gradient
- Chamoattractants for chemotaxis are–Bacterial products, C5a complement protein, leukotrienes and chemokines such as interleukin 8
- Chemoattractants cause receptor activation of leucocytes which cause changes in actin—myosin complex in cell leading to pseudopod formation which helps in locomotion towards site of injury.

PHAGOCYTOSIS

Definition: It is defined as a process by which leucocytes and macrophages secrete enzymes for elimination of microbes.

Steps of phagocytosis

Step I–Recognition and attachment

- Leucocytes and histiocytes recognize microbial particles with the help of receptors on its surface
- Opsonised bacteria are easily recognized and firmly attached by leucocytes.

Step II – Engulfment

- Leucocytes send pseudopods around the microbe and engulf it to form phagosome
- The phagosome binds with lysosome to produce phagolysosome.

Step III–Killing and degradation

- It occurs by 2 mechanisms:
  - *Oxygen dependant H_2O_2:* myeloperoxidase – halide system by which neutrophil granules release myeloperoxidase enzyme which convert H_2O_2 in hydroxyl and hypochlorite free radicals which degrade microbial proteins
  - *Oxygen independent mechanisms:* Neutrophil granules release major basic protein, lactoferrin and lysozymes which activate phospholipase enzyme which degrade phospholipid membrane of bacteria.

CHEMICAL MEDIATORS OF INFLAMMATION

Definition: They are chemical substances synthesized or released which mediate the changes in inflammation.

Functions

Chemotaxis
- C5a complement protein
- Leukotriene B_4
- Chemokines

Vasodilation
- Prostaglandins
- Nitric oxide

Increased vascular permeability
- Histamine, serotonin
- C3a, C5a complement proteins
- Bradykinin
- PAF
- Leukotrienes

Classification

Plasma derived mediators
- Kinin system
- Coagulation system
- Complement system

Cellular mediators

Preformed mediators
- *Histamine* – Source: Mast cells, basophils, platelets
- *Serotonin* – Source: Platelets
- *Lysosomal enzymes* – Source: Neutrophils, Macrophages

Newly synthesized
- *Prostaglandins* – Source: Leucocytes, platelets, endothelial cells
- *Leukotrienes* – Source: Leucocytes
- *Nitric oxide* – Source: Macrophages
- *Cytokines* – Source: Lymphocytes, macrophages, endothelial cells
- *Platelet activating factor (PAF)* – Source: Leucocytes, endothelial cells.

12

CELLULAR MEDIATORS OF INFLAMMATION

Vasoactive amines

- *Histamine*: Released by mast cells, basophils and platelets in response to injury, immune reactions, anaphylatoxins (C3a, C5a), cytokines (IL1, IL8) and cause vasodilation by venular endothelial cell contraction and junctional widening
- *Serotonin*: Released by platelets and have functions similar to histamine.

Arachidonic acid metabolites

- Arachidonic acid on action by 5-lipoxygenase enzyme gives rise to leukotrienes (LT):
  - LTB_4 is involved in chemotaxis
  - LTC_4, D_4, E_4 produce increased vascular permeability, vasoconstriction and bronchoconstriction
- Arachidonic acid on action by 12-lipoxygenase enzyme gives rise to lipoxins (LX)
  - LXA_4 and B_4 cause vasodilation and inhibit neutrophil chemotaxis
- Arachidonic acid on action by cycloxygenase enzyme gives rise to prostaglandins, prostacyclins and thromboxanes:
  - PGD_2, E_2, $F_{2\alpha}$ cause vasodilation and increased vascular permeability
  - Prostacyclin (PGI_2) cause vasodilation and inhibits platelet aggregation
  - Thrombosome A2 (TXA_2) causes vasoconstriction and promotes platelet aggregation.

Nitric oxide

- It is a short acting soluble free radical gas produced by endothelial cells and macrophages
- It causes vascular smooth muscle relaxation and vasodilation especially of venules
- It counteracts platelet aggregation
- It is responsible for killing microbes in activated macrophages
- It also produces reduction in leucocyte adhesion with endothelium.

CELLULAR MEDIATORS OF INFLAMMATION (contd.)

Platelet activating factor (PAF)

- It is chemically acetyl – glyceryl – ether – phosphorylcholine
- It is synthesized by mast cells, platelets, basophils neutrophils, macrophages and endothelial cells
- Functions of PAF are:
  - Vasoconstriction at high concentration
  - Vasodilation and increased venular permeability at low concentration
  - Increased leucocyte adhesion to endothelium
  - Chemotaxis
  - Oxidative burst in phagocytosis.

Cytokines

- Interleukin1 and tumor necrosis factor are two major cytokines involved in inflammation and are synthesized by macrophages in response to microbial infection, immune mediated injury and physical injury
- Functions of cytokines are:
  - Increased leucocytes adhesion to endothelial cells
  - Increased prostacyclin synthesis
  - Increased procoagulant and decreased anticoagulant activity
  - Increased fibroblast proliferation and collagen synthesis
  - Increased acute phase proteins
  - Increased PGE_2 synthesis.

PLASMA DERIVED MEDIATORS OF INFLAMMATION

Complement system

- They are a group of 20 proteins lying in inactive form in plasma
- They are activated by classical pathway, alternate pathway or lectin pathway to form membrane attack complex
- Functions: C3a and C5a cause vasodilation and increased vascular permeability
    - C5a causes neutrophil chemotaxis
    - C3b acts as an opsonin for opsonization of bacteria.

Clotting system

- It is a group of plasma proteins activated by Hageman factor (Factor XIIa)
- Thrombin converts fibrinogen to fibrin which further gives rise to fibrinopeptides which cause increased vascular permeability and enhances neutrophil chemotaxis
- Plasmin causes degradation of fibrin to fibrin split products which cause increased vascular permeability
- Plasmin converts C3 into C3a which is most critical step in complement pathway activation.

Kinin system

- Bradykinin is a vasoactive nanopeptide synthesized by high molecular weight kininogens
- Functions:
    - Vasodilatation
    - Increased vascular permeability
    - Stimulates released of histamine
    - Activates arachidonic acid metabolic pathway
    - Smooth muscle contraction
    - Mediates pain pathway.

CHRONIC INFLAMMATION

Definition: It is an inflammatory process of prolonged duration in which active inflammation, tissue destruction and healing are proceeding simultaneously **(Fig. 8)**.

Causes

- Chronic persistent infections
- Prolonged toxin exposure e.g. silica
- Autoimmune reactions.

Specialized type

Chronic granulomatous inflammation (Fig. 4)

- It is a type of inflammation characterized by accumulation of activated macrophages which have epithelial cell-like appearance
- Examples: Tuberculosis, leprosy, fungal infection, cat scatch disease, sarcoidosis, berryliosis.

Steps

I – Mononuclear cell infiltration

- Inflammatory focus in infiltrated by macrophages, lymphocytes and plasma cells
- Activated macrophages release toxic O_2 species and proteases which cause tissue and pathogen destruction
- They also release factors which activate arachidonic acid metabolite pathway, nitric oxide and neutrophil chemotaxis.

II – Tissue destruction

- Destruction of tissue occurs due to toxins released by microbes and mediators released by mononuclear cells invading the site.

III – Healing by fibrosis

- Activated macrophages release certain growth factors like platelet derived growth factor (PDGF), fibroblast growth factor (FGF) and vascular endothelial growth factor (VEGF) which promotes fibrosis and angiogenesis leading to healing by fibrosis.

16

WOUND HEALING

Factors affecting wound healing

- *Local factors*:
  - Blood supply
  - Local infection
  - Hematoma
  - Foreign body
  - Mechanical stress
  - Necrosis
  - Type of tissue
  - Nerve supply
- *Systemic factors*:
  - Age
  - Anemia
  - Drugs
  - Collagen genetic diseases
  - Diabetes mellitus
  - Malnutrition
  - Obesity
  - Septicemia
  - Uremia
  - Vitamin C deficiency
  - Zinc, copper deficiency.

Complications

- Deficient scar formation
- Keloid and hypertrophic scar
- Contractures: Due to excessive wound contraction.

Types

- Healing by primary intention (apposed edges)
  - Neutrophilic infiltration for 24–48 hrs
  - Neutrophils replaced by macrophages in 3 days
  - Granulation tissue formation by 5 days
  - Fibroblast proliferation and initiation of fibrosis by 7–10 days
  - Fibrous union by 1 week
- Healing by secondary intention (unopposed edges)
  - Larger fibrin clot and denser inflammation
  - Larger amount of granulation tissue formation
  - Severe wound contraction and scar formation.

Steps

Step I – Thrombosis

- A clot referred as a scab forms a barrier on wound preventing microbial invasion
- Factors involved: Factor XIIIa, transforming growth factor (TGF) α and β, PDGF
- Source: Plasma, platelets.

Step II – Inflammation

- Neutrophils infiltrate the wound to remove microbes and necrotic debris
- Plasma derived fibronectin and neutrophil debris act as chemoattractants for macrophages and fibroblasts
- Macrophages eat neutrophil debris and release factors for fibrogenesis and angiogenesis
- Factor involved: TGF-β
- Source: Neutrophil.

WOUND HEALING (contd.)

Steps (contd.)

Step III – Granulation tissue formation

- It is the transient specialized organ of repair
- It is composed of:
    - Erythrocytes and fibroblasts followed by
    - Single cell lined capillaries surrounded by
    - Fibroblasts and macrophages
- Factor involved: FGF, TGF-β
- Source: Macrophages, fibroblasts.

Step IV – Fibroblast proliferation and matrix accumulation

- 2 – 3 days after injury, fibroblasts start secreting collagen especially type III
- About 5 – 7 days, collagen type I is formed which imparts tensile strength to wound
- Source – Macrophages, fibroblasts.

Step V – Angiogenesis

- It occurs either from endothelial precursor cells or angioblasts which travel from basement membrane to inflammation site where they transform into endothelial cells, pericytes and smooth muscle cells of blood vessel
- It also occurs from previously present vessels near the site by degradation of basement membrane and proliferation of endothelial cells
- Factors involved: VEGF
- Source: Macrophage, monocyte.

Step VI – Wound contraction

- It is done by specialized type of fibroblasts called myofibroblasts (MF)
- MFs contain actin which has contractile abilities
- Multiple MFs form tight junctions and contract leading to wound contraction
- Factors involved: TGF-β_1, TGF-β_2
- Source: Platelets, macrophages, monocytes, fibroblasts.

Step VII – Accretion of tensile strength and remodelling

- Tensile strength is restored by cross linking of collagen fibres
- Remodelling occurs as wound site devascularises
- Factors involved: PDGF, FGF, matrix metalloproteinases, tissue inhibitor of metalloproteinases
- Source: Platelets, fibroblasts, capillaries.

EDEMA

Definition: It is defined as the presence of excess fluid in the interstitial spaces of the body.

Types:
- Localized edema
- Generalized edema (Anasarca)

Pathophysiology

- Congestive cardiac failure → Increased hydrostatic capillary pressure → Increased interstitial fluid
- Congestive cardiac failure → Decreased cardiac output
- Decreased plasma oncotic pressure → Decrease blood volume → Decreased cardiac output
- Decreased cardiac output → Decreased effective arterial volume → Increased renin → Increased aldosterone → Increase renal Sodium and H_2O
- Renal insufficiency → Increase renal Sodium and H_2O
- Increase renal Sodium and H_2O → Increased plasma volume → Increased interstitial fluid → Edema

Etiopathogenesis: Based on pathophysiology, causes are:

- Increased hydrostatic pressure
  - Arteriolar dilation
    - Heat
    - Inflammation
  - Impaired venous return
    - Congestive cardiac failure
    - Cirrhosis
    - Venous thrombosis
    - Postural inactivity
  - Hypervolemia
    - Renal insufficiency
- Decreased plasma oncotic pressure
  - Hypoproteinemia
    - Nephrotic syndrome
    - Cirrhosis
    - Protein losing gastroenteropathy
    - Malnutrition
  - Increased capillary permeability
    - Inflammation
    - Burns
- Lymphatic obstruction
  - Neoplasia
  - Post-surgery
  - Post-irradiation
  - Filariasis

HYPEREMIA

Definition: It is defined as an active process of augmented supply of blood to an organ.

Causes

- Exercise
- Anemia
- Transient ischemia
- Inflammation

CONGESTION

Definition: It is a passive process of engorgement of an organ with venous blood.

Causes

- Left heart failure
- Right heart failure
- Isolated venous obstruction secondary to thrombosis, tumor and emboli.

Morphology

Gross morphology

- In right heart failure, congestion occurs in liver and spleen
- In left heart failure, congestion occurs in lung
- Grossly, the organ is hemorrhagic and wet on cut surface; in liver, alternate pale and dark bands formed giving it an appearance of nutmeg.

Microscopy

- In chronic venous congestion of lung, alveolar septae are thick and fibrotic with hemosiderin laden alveolar macrophages called heart failure cells in alveoli **(Fig. 9)**
- In chronic venous congestion of liver, there is centrilobular necrosis and hemorrhage with hemosiderin laden macrophages **(Fig. 10 and Image F)**
- In chronic venous congestion spleen, there is increased fibrotic bands with iron and calcium containing fibrotic foci (Gamma – Gandy bodies) seen along with multiple areas of hemorrhage.

THROMBOSIS

Definition: It refers to formation of a thrombus which is defined as an aggregate of coagulated blood containing platelets, fibrin and entrapped cells with in a vascular lumen **(Fig. 11).**

Pathogenesis: It involves principally 3 factors (Virchow triad):

- Endothelial damage – usually by atherosclerosis
- Alterations in blood flow –
- Increased coagulability of blood – causes of hypercoagulable blood includes:
  - Mutations in factor V, prothrombin gene
  - Antithrombin, protein C and S deficiency
  - Prolonged bedrest
  - Myocardial infarction
  - Cancer
  - Disseminated intravascular coagulation
  - Prosthetic heart valves
  - Anti-phospholipid antibody syndrome
  - Trauma and burns
  - Smoking.

Sequelae

- Propagation
- Embolization
- Lysis
- Organization and Recanalization

Morphology

- Thrombi occur in any part of cardiovascular system
- Based on location, they are of 2 types.

Arterial thrombus

- They begin at site of endothelial injury or turbulence
- They develop retrograde from point of attachment
- They are pale, firm and grey white
- Lines of Zahn are prominent
- Embolization is less common
- Sites: Coronary, cerebral and femoral artery.

Venous thrombosis

- They occur in site of thrombosis
- The develop antegrade along the flow of blood
- They contains more erythrocytes and are red
- Lines of Zahn are not very apparent
- Emboli formation is common
- Sites: Deep veins of legs, periprostatic and ovarian plexus.

EMBOLISM

Definition: It is defined as the passage through venous or arterial circulation of any material capable of lodging in a blood vessel and causing obstruction.

Types

Systemic thromboembolism

- Heart is most common source of arterial thromboemboli
- Most common sites of emboli:
  - Brain
  - Intestine
  - Lower extremity
  - Kidney
  - Heart
- Causes:
  - Left ventricular wall myocardial infarction
  - Aortic aneurysm
  - Vascular atherosclerosis

Amniotic fluid embolism

- It refers to the entry of amniotic fluid containing fetal cells and debris in maternal circulation through uterine and cervical veins.
- Clinical manifestations:
  - Cyanosis
  - Dyspnea
  - Shock
  - Coma
  - Disseminated intravascular coagulation
  - Acute respiratory distress syndrome.

Pulmonary thromboembolism

- It occurs in 1 – 2 % of postoperative patients over 40 years of age
- Site of origin:
  - Iliofemoral veins (90%)
  - Pelvic venous plexus
  - Right side of heart
- Acute pulmonary embolism has following variable manifestations:
  - Asymptomatic small pulmonary emboli
  - Transient dyspnea and tachypnea
  - Pulmonary infarction with pleuritis and pleural effusion
  - Cardivascular collapse with sudden death.

EMBOLISM (contd.) → **Types (contd.)**

Air embolism

- 100 cc of air is required to produce clinical manifestation of air emboli
- Causes:
  - Trauma
  - Thoracocentesis
  - Puncture of great veins during invasive procedure
  - Under water workers
  - Scuba divers
- In last 2 causes, the disease is called decompression sickness and occurs due to sudden change in pressure due to sudden ascent from deeper water
- Acute decompression sickness is known as bends and chokes
  - Bends is characterized by myalgia and arthralgia owing to small blood vessel obstruction
  - Chokes is respiratory distress due to edema and hemorrhage in lung
- Chronic decompression sickness is called as Caisson disease and presents with multiple ischemic necrotic foci in bones and skeletal muscles.

Fat embolism

- It refers to entry of emboli of fatty marrow into damaged blood vessels following trauma to fat containing tissue
- It occurs in most cases of trauma but clinically presents in 10% cases
- Symptoms develop 1 – 3 days after trauma
- Clinical manifestations:
  - Tachypnea
  - Dyspnea
  - Mental changes due to cerebral edema
  - Thrombocytopenia
  - Petechiae

INFARCTION

Definition: It is defined as the process by which ischemic coagulative necrosis develops in an area distal to occlusion of an end artery or proximal to occlusion of its venous drainage.

Etiopathogenesis

- Factors affecting the development of an infarct are:
  - *Nature of blood supply* : Organs with dual blood supply are resistant to infarction as compared to organs with single blood supply
  - *Rate of development of occlusion*: Slower the occlusion of blood vessel, lesser is the risk of infarction
  - *Organs capability to tolerate hypoxia*: Certain organs like brain and heart are vulnerable to hypoxia as compared to other organs like liver and develop faster infarcts
  - *Oxygen content of blood.*

Morphology

- Infarcts are classified based on color into:
  - Red infarcts (Hemorrhagic)
  - White infarcts (Anemic)
- Infarcts are classified based on microbial infection into:
  - Septic infarct
  - Bland infarct

Red infarcts (Fig. 12)

- They occur in following settings:
  - When tissue is loose and spongy
  - Due to venous occlusion of an organ
  - Tissue with dual blood supply
- They occur in small intestine and brain
- Grossly, they have ill-defined margins and grey-red to purple in colour.

White infarcts (Fig. 13 and Image A)

- The occur in following settings:
  - The tissues are firm and solid
  - Due to arterial occlusion of organ
  - Organs with end arterial circulation
- They are seen in heart, spleen and kidney
- Grossly, they are wedge shaped, pale coloured with well-defined margins and have an apex and base.

Definition: It is defined as a condition of profound hemodynamic and metabolic disturbance characterized by failure of circulating system to maintain apt blood supply to microcirculation with consequent inadequate perfusion of vital organs.

SHOCK

Stages of shock: It is divided into 3 stages:

- *Non-progressive phase*
- *Progressive stage* characterized by tissue hypoperfusion and onset of metabolic imbalances
- *Irreversible stage*

Morphology: Shock is characterized by multiorgan dysfunction and changes seen are:

- Brain – Ischemic encephalopathy ensues
- Heart – Coagulative necrosis and subendocardial hemorrhages seen
- Kidneys – Acute tubular necrosis seen
- Lungs – Diffuse alveolar damage
- GIT – Diffuse mucosal hemorrhages all over the gut
- Liver – Marked centrilobular congestion and necrosis noted.

Pathogenesis: Based on various pathogenic causes, shock is classified into 5 groups:

- *Cardiogenic shock*: It is caused by myocardial pump failure and is seen in:
    - Myocardial infarction
    - Myocarditis
    - Cardiac tamponade
    - Pulmonary embolism
- *Hypovolemic shock*: It is caused by decrease in blood or plasma volume caused by fluid loss and is seen in:
    - Hemorrhage
    - Burns
    - Dehydration
    - Diarrhea
- *Anaphylactic shock*: It occurs due to vasodilation caused by type I hypersensitivity reaction
- *Neurogenic shock*: It occurs due to acute brain injury causing vasomotor centre damage leading to vasodilation and decreased effective circulatory volume
- *Septic shock*: Gram-negative organism septicemia is most common cause of septic shock:
    - Endotoxin of organism contains lipopolysaccharide which has lipid A which binds with lipopolysaccharide binding protein in circulation
    - The complex then binds CD14 receptor on macrophage/monocytes leading to secretion of various mediators like tumor necrosis factor, interleukin1, 6, 8, 12 and nitric oxide.
    - There mediators cause vasodilation and severe cardiovascular compressive and shock.

AUTOSOMAL CHROMOSOMAL DISORDERS

Down syndrome

- Most common chromosomal disorder characterized by trisomy of chromosome 21
- It is seen in 1 in every 700 child births and is major cause of mental retardation
- Karyotype – 47, XX + 21
- Clinical features:
  - Mental retardation
  - Flat facies and epicanthic folds
  - Simian crease on palms
  - Abundant neck skin
  - Congenital heart defects– Ventricular septal defect and atrial septal defect
  - Intestinal stenosis
  - Umbilical hernia
  - Hypotonia
  - Gap between Ist and IInd toe.

Patau syndrome

- It is a chromosomal syndrome characterized by trisomy of chromosome 13.
- It is seen in 1 in every 15000 childbirths
- Karyotype – 47, XX + 13
- Clinical features:
  - Microcephaly
  - Mental retardation
  - Microphthalmia
  - Polydactyly
  - Cleft lip and palate
  - Cardiac defects
  - Renal defects
  - Umbilical hernia
  - Rocker bottom feet.

Edward syndrome

- It is a chromosomal disorder characterized by trisomy of chromosome 18
- It is seen in 1 in every 7000 childbirths
- Karyotype – 47, XX + 18
- Clinical features:
  - Prominent occiput
  - Mental retardation
  - Micrognathia
  - Low set ears
  - Short neck
  - Overlapping fingers
  - Renal malformations – Horse shoe kidney
  - Limited hip abduction
  - Rocker bottom foot.

SEX CHROMOSOMAL DISORDERS

Turner syndrome

- It is a spectrum of abnormalities occurring in a phenotypic female that results from presence of complete or partial monosomy of X-chromosome.
- It occurs in 1 in 3000 female childbirths
- Karyotype – 45 + XO
- Clinical features:
    - Short stature
    - Low posterior hairline
    - Webbing of neck
    - Broad chest and widely spaced nipples
    - Coarctation of arota
    - Cubitus valgus
    - Pigmented nevi
    - Streaked ovary
    - Infertility
    - Amenorrhea
    - Lymphedema at birth

Lyon hypothesis

- Proposed by Lyon in 1961
- The hypothesis has 4 tenets –
    - Only one X-chromosome is active
    - Other X-chromosome undergoes heteropyknosis and becomes inactive
    - Inactivation occurs randomly in all cells at blastocyst stage by 16th day of embryonic life
    - Inactivation of same X-chromosome persist in all cells derived from each precursor cell.

Klinefelter's syndrome

- It is a testicular dysgenesis related to presence of excess of one or more X-chromosome in excess of normal XY-genotype
- It is seen in 1 in 500 livebirths
- Karyotype – 47, XXY
- Clinical features:
    - Hypogonadism at puberty
    - Increased length of bones between soles and pubic bone
    - Small penis
    - Lack of secondary sexual characteristics like deep voice, beard and male distribution of pubic hairs
    - Gynecomastia
    - Low IQ
    - Reduced spermatogenesis
    - Associated breast cancer
    - Associated germ cell tumor
    - Associated with systemic lupus erythematosus
    - Reduced testosterone levels
    - Increased plasma estradiol levels
    - Increased follicular stimulating hormone levels.

TYPE I HYPERSENSITIVITY (ANAPHYLAXIS)

Definition: It is a fast developing immune reaction which occurs within minutes of exposure of antigen to the antibodies bound to mast cells in individuals previously sensitized to the antigen.

Mechanism

Ist exposure to antigen

↓

Antigen presenting cells present antigen to T_H2 helper T-cells

↓

T_H2 helper T-cells release interleukin (IL) 4 which activates B cells to produce immunoglobulin E, IL3 and IL5 which activate eosinophils

↓

IgE released from B cells actively bind to Fc receptor on mast cells and basophils

↓

On re-exposure to antigen, mast cells undergo degranulation and release primary and secondary mediators

Secondary mediators are

- Leukotrienes C4 and D4 which are strong spasmogenic agents
- Prostaglandin D2 causes bronchospasm and increased mucus secretion
- Platelet activating factor which causes bronchospasm, increased vascular permeability, vasodilation and increased release of histamine.

Primary mediators are

- Histamine – which cause smooth muscle contraction, increased secretion from glands and increased vascular permeability
- Proteases and acid hydrolases cause tissue degradation
- Proteoglycans – store mediators in granules.

Examples

- Hay fever
- Asthma
- Urticaria
- Atopy
- Anaphylaxis

TYPE II HYPERSENSITIVITY (ANTIBODY MEDIATED HYPERSENSITIVITY)

Definition: It is defined as a type of hypersensitivity which is mediated by IgM or IgG antibodies directed against fixed antigen in tissues located on cell surface or extracellular matrix.

Mechanism: There are 3 main mechanisms:

- Opsonization and complement mediated phagocytosis:

  The target cells are coated with antibodies
  ↓
  This leads to activation of complement
  ↓
  C3b binds with antibody bound cells
  ↓
  C3b receptor of phagocytes detect C3b and leads to phagocytosis

- Complement and Fc receptor mediated inflammation:

  Antibodies are bound to extracellular matrix
  ↓
  These antibodies activate complement and produce C5a and C3a
  ↓
  C5a recruits and activate neutrophils and monocytes
  ↓
  Leucocytes release mediators and damage tissue

- Antibody mediated cellular dysfunction:

  Antibodies bind to receptors on cell surface
  ↓
  They dysregulate function of cell.

Examples

- Autoimmune hemolytic anemia
- Autoimmune thrombocytopenic purpura
- Wegener granulomatosis
- Goodpasture's syndrome
- Rheumatic fever
- Myasthenia gravis
- Grave disease
- Insulin dependent diabetes mellitus
- Pernicious anemia.

Definition: It is characterized by immune complex deposition, complement fixation and localized inflammation which occurs when IgG or IgM and rarely IgA antibody binds with circulating or fixed antigen located in a tissue.

TYPE III HYPERSENSITIVITY (IMMUNE COMPLEX HYPERSENSITIVITY)

Examples

- Serum sickness
- Arthus reaction
- Septic arthritis
- Post-streptococcal glomerulonephritis
- Polyarteritis nodosa
- Systemic lupus erythematosus

Mechanism

Formation of antigen – antibody complex in circulation

↓

Fixation of immune complex in tissues

↓

- Activation of neutrophils and monocytes due to thin Fc receptor binding with immune complexes and causing activation of phagocytes leading to release of lysosomal enzymes to cause tissue damage
- Activation of complement which produce neutrophils and macrophage chemotactic factors like C5a and anaphylatoxins like C3a and C5a which increases vascular permeability
- Platelet aggregation and activation of factor XII leads to microthrombi formation in blood vessels causing ischemic vasculitis leading to tissue damage

TYPE IV HYPERSENSITIVITY (DELAYED TYPE CELL MEDIATED HYPERSENSITIVITY)

Definition: It refers to an antigen elicited cellular immune reaction that results in tissue damage and does not require participation of antibodies and includes reaction mediated by CD4 + T-cells and CD8 + T-cells.

Examples
- Rheumatoid arthritis
- Tuberculosis
- Guillain Barre syndrome
- Contact dermatitis
- Multiple sclerosis

Mechanism

- Delayed type hypersensitivity (CD4 + T-cell-mediated) mechanism:

Antigen binds with antigen presenting cells

↓

Cell receptor on CD4 + T-cells recognize site on antigen presenting cell

↓

CD4 + T-cells is activated and converted to T_H1 helper T-cells under the effect of IL12 secreted by antigen presenting cell

↓

T_H1 helper T-cells secrete tumor necrosis factor (TNF), interferon γ and IL2

↓

TNF causes secretion of prostacyclins and activation of adhesion molecules on macrophages and lymphocytes.

IFNγ is powerful macrophage activator which enhances its phagocytic activity, transforms it to epithelioid cells and promotes secretion of PDGF which stimulate fibrosis.

IL2 cause autocrine proliferation of CD4+ T-cells.

- Direct cell cytotoxicity (CD8 + T-cell-mediated) mechanism:

Antigen presenting cells (APC) bind with antibody

↓

CD8 + T-cell recognize APC with major histocompatibility complex molecule

↓

CD8 + T-cell-activated to cytotoxic CD8 + T-cell

↓

Destruction of APC.

SYSTEMIC LUPUS ERYTHEMATOSUS

Definition: It is defined as a chronic multisystem, autoimmune inflammatory disease that involves any organ but characteristically involves kidney, joints, serous membranes and skin.

Etiopathogenesis: Certain factors are implicated in causation of this autoimmune disorder.

Viral infection especially Epstein-Barr virus, excess of estrogen, drugs like procainamide and genetic predisposition

↓

Loss of immune tolerance | Acquired sensitivity to autoantigens

↓

Autoreactive CD4 + T-cells

↓

Polyclonal B-cell hyperreactivity

↓

Autoantibody production like antinuclear antibody (ANA) and anti-dsDNA antibody

↓

Immune complex formation in blood and tissues

↓

Tissue injury

- Glomerulonephritis
- Vasculitis
- Serositis
- Arthritis

SYSTEMIC LUPUS ERYTHEMATOSUS (contd.)

Morphology

- Multisystem involvement caused by vasculitis of blood vessel supplying the organ.

Pulmonary lesions

- Lesions in lung are:
  - Pleuritis
  - Pleural effusion
  - Alveolitis

Joint lesions

- Non-erosive synovitis of joints characterized histologically by neutrophilic infiltration of synovium.

Skin lesions

- Butterfly erythema on face involving cheek and bridge of nose.
- Similar lesions seen anywhere on skin
- Microscopically, liquefactive degeneration of basal cells with edema at dermoepidermal junction and mononuclear inflammation in dermis.

Renal lesions

- Lesions in kidney are classified into 5 groups:
  - Minimal abnormality (class I)
  - Mesangial lupus glomerulonephritis (class II)
  - Focal proliferative glomerulonephritis (class III)
  - Diffuse proliferative glomerulonephritis (class IV)
  - Membranoproliferative glomerulonephritis (class V)

Cardiovascular lesions

- Lesions in heart include:
  - Pericarditis
  - Myocarditis
  - Non-bacterial verrucous endocarditis.

Definition: It is a group of diverse extracellular protein deposits which have common morphological characteristic affinity for specialized dyes and a characteristic appearance under polarized light.

Classification

- It is classified into 2 groups based on localization of amyloid:
  - *Localized amyloidosis*
  - *Systemic amyloidosis*: Based on etiology it is classified into:
    - Primary amyloidosis: It is seen in association with immunocyte dyscrasias and characterized by deposition of AL protein
    - Secondary amyloidosis: It is seen in association with systemic diseases and characterized by deposition of AA protein.

Physical nature of amyloid

- It is an amorphous, hyaline, eosinophilic extracellular substance **(Fig. 14)** and is physically composed of fibrils of indefinite length and 7.5–10 nm diameter arranged in a β-pleated sheet.

AMYLOIDOSIS

Classification table

Clinicopathological entity	Amyloid protein deposited
Systemic amyloidosis	
• Primary amyloidosis	AL
• Secondary amyloidosis	AA
• Hemodialysis associated amyloidosis	$A\beta_2$ m
• Familial amyloidotic polyneuropathy	ATTR
• Systemic senile amyloidosis	ATTR
• Familial mediterranean fever	AA
Localized amyloidosis	
• Senile cerebral amyloidosis	Aβ
• Senile cardiac amyloidosis	AANF
• Medullary thyroid carcinoma	Acal

Stains for amyloid

- It stains red with Congo red dye and gives apple green birefringence under polarized light
- It also stains with thioflavin T, alcian blue and specific antibodies
- It stains yellow to brown with Von Gieson stain
- In fresh tissue, amyloid stains brown with Lugol iodine which converts to blue on treatment with 10% sulphuric acid.

AMYLOIDOSIS (contd.)

Etiopathogenesis

- In primary amyloidosis, plasma cells secrete immunoglobulin light chains which undergo limited proteolysis to AL and deposited in tissues
- In secondary amyloidosis, chronic inflammation leads to macrophage activation which secrete interleukins IL1 and 6 which activates hepatocytes to secrete SAA proteins which undergo partial proteolysis to AA proteins and accumulated in tissue
- In some cases, proteins are misfolded, become insoluble and accumulated in tissues as small oligomers.

Morphology

Gross morphology

- *Kidney*: It is mildly enlarged and has waxy cut surface appearance
- *Spleen*: It is moderate to markedly enlarged
- *Liver*: It is moderately enlarged and has waxy cut surface
- *Heart*: It is mildly enlarged and firm in consistency.

Microscopy

- *Kidney*: Amyloid is primarily deposited in glomeruli and rarely in interstitium and renal blood vessels **(Fig. 14)**
- *Spleen*:
  - Sago spleen – Amyloid is deposited in splenic follicles
  - Lardaceous spleen – Amyloid is deposited in splenic sinuses in red pulp
- *Liver*: Amyloid is first deposited in space of Disse followed by involvement of sinuses and hepatocytes
- *Heart*: Amyloid is deposited in subendocardium and interstitial tissue between myocardial fibres.

NEOPLASM

Definition: It is defined as an abnormal mass of tissue which has uncoordinated and excessive growth potential much higher than its normal tissue of origin.

Types

Malignant neoplasm (Figs 36, 39, 43, 45 and 46)
- Tumor is well to poorly differentiated with mild to severe degree of anaplasia
- The tumor growth is rapid with plenty of mitoses seen
- The tumor is locally invasive and erodes into the surrounding tissue
- Metastasis is often seen; poor the differentiation, higher the incidence of metastasis.

Benign neoplasm (Figs 15, 16, 17 and 18)
- Tumor is well-differentiated with tumor cells resembling tissue of origin with minimal to no anaplasia
- Tumors are slow growing which may regress in size and have low mitotic activity
- Tumor mass is well-defined and doesn’t invade local surrounding tissue
- Benign tumors do not metastasize to distant sites.

METASTASIS

Definition: It is defined as transfer of malignant cells from one site to another site not directly connected to tumor site.

Mechanism

- Steps of metastasis are:
  - Invasion of basement membrane underlying tumor
  - Tumor cell movement through extracellular matrix
  - Invasion into vascular or lymphatic channel
  - Survival and arrest within circulation
  - Exit from circulation at new site
  - Tumor homing, angiogenesis and growth
- Normal cells are bound to each other with E-cadherin and catenin molecules; E-cadherin expression is lost in most cancers leading to loosening of tumor cells
- Tumor cells bind with basement membrane laminin and fibronectin
- Tumor cells release matrix metalloproteinases 9 and 2 which cause degradation of basement membrane, extracellular matrix and vascular basement membrane
- Tumor cells adhere to each other and to blood cells in circulation and form tumor emboli
- CD44 receptors on tumor emboli helps in homing at new site as CD44 on T-lymphocytes binds with hyaluronate
- The tumor emboli pierce the vessel and reach the site where tumor cells secrete VEGF and bFGF which helps in development of vascular supply within tumor.

METASTASIS (contd.)

Types

- Based on the pathways of spread, metastasis is of three main types.

Serous cavity metastasis

- Malignant tumors that arise in organs adjacent to serous cavity produce metastasis due to shedding of tumor cells in them
- Gastrointestinal tract and ovarian tumors metastasize in peritoneal cavity
- Lung tumors metastasize in pleural space.

Hematogenous metastasis

- It is common in sarcomas but is also seen in carcinomas
- Cancer cells commonly invade capillaries and vessels
- Arteries and arterioles are resistant to invasion
- Most abdominal tumors invade portal vein and produce hepatic metastasis
- Other tumors invade systemic veins and cause lung metastasis.

Lymphatic metastasis (Fig. 19)

- It is a preferential method of metastasis in carcinomas but sarcomas may also follow this route
- Tumor doesn't contain lymphatics thus, invade lymph capillaries in adjacent normal tissue
- Metastasis occur in lymphatic drainage site
- It is faster as compared to hematogenous metastasis as small lymph capillaries lack basement membrane.

MOLECULAR BASIS OF CARCINOGENESIS

Molecular genetic changes occurring in cancers are as follows:

- Oncogene activation
- Antioncogene suppression
- Impairment of DNA repair genes
- Inhibition of apoptotic genes
- Overexpression of telomerase.

Oncogene activation

- Oncogenes are overactive counterpart of normal protooncogenes
- Activation of protooncogenes with their over expression occurs by 3 mechanisms:
  - Mutation in protooncogene
  - Activation by translocation
  - Activation by gene amplification
- Oncogenes are classified into 5 groups:
  - Growth factors, e.g. TGFα overexpression in hepatocellular carcinoma and gliomas
  - Growth factor receptors, e.g. Her – 2/neu amplification in breast carcinoma
  - Signal transducer genes, e.g. point mutation in RAS gene in colon, lung and pancreatic cancers
  - Nuclear regulatory genes, e.g. c – MYC gene translocation in Burkitt lymphoma
  - Cell cycle regulator genes, e.g. cyclin D and E overexpression in carcinoma breast.

Antioncogene suppression

- Tumor supressor genes are inhibited by somatic or germ line mutation to cause cancers
- Antioncogenes are classified into 5 groups based on the location of their proteins in cell:
  - Cell surface, e.g. E-cadherin inhibited in gastric carcinoma
  - Inner surface of plasma membrane, e.g. NF1 gene mutation in neuroblastoma and neurofibromatosis type 1
  - Cytoskeleton, e.g. NF2 gene mutation in neurofibromatosis type 2, schwanomma and meningioma
  - Cytosol, e.g. PTEN mutation in endometrial carcinoma
  - Nucleus, e.g. p53 mutation in most cancers, RB gene mutation in retinoblastoma and osteosarcoma.

MOLECULAR BASIS OF CARCINOGENESIS (contd.)

Ielomerase overexpression

- The normal cell ages due to shortening of telomeres in their chromosomes
- In certain tumors, telomerase gene is activated producing telomerase enzyme which inhibit shortening of telomeres and cause increased life of tumor cells.

Impairment of DNA repair genes

- DNA repair genes also known as caretaker genes remove the base pair mutations which occur due to assault of mutagenic agents such as radiation, oxidative stress and chemicals, e.g. BRCA1 and BRCA2 gene mutation in familial breast and ovarian cancers
- Disorders with DNA repair gene abnormality e.g. ataxia telangiectasia, xeroderma pigmentosum and Bloom syndrome make the patients very vulnerable to multiple cancers.

Inhibition of apoptosis

- In development of tumor, cells learn to evade apoptosis to live a longer life
- There are certain apoptotic and antiapoptotic genes interplaying in a cell
- Bcl-2 is an antiapoptotic gene which is overexpressed in many B-cell lymphomas
- p53 activates transcription of apoptotic genes like Bak; inactivation of p53 inhibits apoptosis indirectly by inhibition of apoptotic gene transcription.

VIRAL CARCINOGENESIS

- Certain viruses have ability to cause cancers in humans and are classified into 2 groups:
  - DNA oncogenic virus
  - RNA oncogenic virus

RNA oncogenic viral oncogenesis

- Few RNA viruses have ability to induce cancers, e.g. human T-cell leukemia virus type I.

Human T-cell leukemia viral carcinogenesis

- It causes endemic T-cell leukemia and lymphomas by its TAX gene which causes host gene activation causing T-cell proliferation.

DNA oncogenic viral carcinogenesis

- Certain DNA viruses have the ability to induce cancers in humans
  - Human papilloma virus (HPV)
  - Epstein Barr virus (EBV)
  - Hepatitis B virus

EBV induced carcinogenesis

- EBV is involved in causation of African type Burkitt lymphoma, nasopharyngeal carcinoma and some cases of Hodgkin lymphoma
- EBV infects B-lymphocytes and nasopharyngeal epithelial cells
- EBV binds with CD20 receptor to enter B-lymphocyte cell and binds with nucleus as episome
- EBV releases certain proteins like LMP1 (latent membrane protein1) which activates signal transduction pathway thereby, enhancing B-cell survival and proliferation
- EBV derived EBNA-2 gene activates cyclin D gene in host cells causing cell proliferation.

Hepatitis B virus induced carcinogenesis

- Hepatitis B virus is associated with hepatocellular carcinoma
- HBV causes liver cell injury which leads to rapid proliferation due to which hepatocytes are prone to genetic damage
- HBV induces HBX protein which causes activation of protooncogenes such as insulin like growth factor1 (IGF1) gene and IGF1 receptor gene
- HBX protein binds with p53 and inhibits its cell proliferation activity.

HPV induced carcinogenesis

- High-risk HPV, i.e. HPV16, 18, 31, 33 and 55 are found in association with squamous cell carcinoma in 80 – 90% cases
- The viral DNA of HPV binds with human cell nuclear genome at its E1/E2 opening site
- The E6 and E7 protein of viral DNA binds with p53 gene and enhances its degradation causing a block in apoptosis
- The E7 protein inhibits p21 which is a cell cycle inhibitor and retinoblastoma (RB) gene which removes the growth arrest signal produced by RB protein.

CHEMICAL CARCINOGENESIS

Definition: It is defined as induction of cancer in human by carcinogenic chemicals.

Steps

- Chemical carcinogenesis is a 4 step process:
  - *Initiation*: In this step, initiator chemical cause mutation in single cell
  - *Promotion*: Under influence of certain promoter chemicals, the initiated cell undergoes clonal expansion
  - *Progression*: In this stage, adequate mutations have occurred in cell imparting it immortality and autonomous growth
  - *Cancer formation*: Finally, the cells develop capacity to invade and metastasize.

Carcinogens

- *Polycycline aromatic hydrocarbons*: They require metabolic activation and are produced by cigarette smoke; they are implicated in majority of human cancers, e.g. lung and bladder carcinoma
- *Alkylating agents*: They are activation independent and are used as anticancer drugs, e.g. cyclophosphamide, busulfan etc. (While they treat one cancer, they induce other cancers like lymphomas and leukemias.)
- *Aflatoxin*: It is a mycotoxin produced by *Aspergillus flavus* and produce hepatocellular carcinoma
- *Azo dyes*: They are metabolized in liver and induce hepatocellular and urinary bladder carcinoma
- *Nitrosamines*: They are implicated in gastric carcinoma.

RADIATION CARCINOGENESIS

- Radiant energy being a high source of energy causes severe mutations in cell nucleus inducing various cancers
- Most potent forms of radiation causing cancers are:
    - Non-ionizing radiation, i.e. ultraviolet (UV) rays
    - Ionising radiation, i.e. elctromagnetic radiation (X-rays, γ-rays) and particulate radiation (α-particles, β-particles).

Ultraviolet rays induced carcinogenesis

- Ultraviolet rays induce cancers of skin, i.e., basal cell carcinoma, melanoma and squamous cell carcinoma
- UVB rays with wavelength of 280 – 320 nm are most potent mutagenic rays
- UVB rays induce carcinogenicity by formation of pyrimidine dimers in DNA and inhibition of nucleotide excision repair pathways of DNA repair
- Ultraviolet rays also induce mutation in oncogenes like RAS and antioncogenes like p53.

Ionising radiation carcinogenesis

- Miners of radioactive mines have high incidence of lung carcinoma
- Radiation exposure in atomic bomb survivors of japan developed leukamias, breast, colon, thyroid and lung cancers
- Residents of Marshall island who were exposed to hydrogen bomb developed cancers in thyroid
- Ionising radiation induced DNA mutations by altering the valencies of elements in purine and pyrimidine dimers.

PARANEOPLASTIC SYNDROMES

Definition: It is defined as a syndrome occurring in a cancer which cannot be explained by metastasis of tumor or by hormones elaborated by the tissue of origin of tumor.

Types

Neurological paraneoplastic syndromes

- Subacute motor neuropathy – seen in association with lymphomas
- Amyotrophic lateral sclerosis – seen in association with carcinoma in 10% patients
- Autonomic neuropathy – seen in small cell carcinoma of lung
- Sensorimotor neuropathy – seen in many cancers.

Muscular paraneoplastic syndromes

- Myasthenia – seen in bronchogenic carcinoma
- Eaton Lambert syndrome – seen in thymomas.

Cutaneous paraneoplastic syndromes

- Acanthosis nigricans – 90% cases of it have cancer of stomach, lung and uterus
- Exfoliative dermatitis – seen in non-Hodgkin and Hodgkin lymphomas
- Dermatomyositis – seen in bronchogenic and breast carcinoma.

Endocrine paraneoplastic syndromes

- Carcinoid syndrome – due to serotonin in bronchial carcinoid, pancreatic and gastric carcinoma
- Syndrome of inappropriate antidiuretic hormone (SIADH) – seen in small cell carcinoma of lung
- Cushing syndrome – due to adrenocorticotropic hormone (ACTH) seen in small cell carcinoma of lung
- Hypercalcemia – due to parathormone related protein in breast carcinoma, renal carcinoma and lung squamous cell carcinoma
- Hypoglycemia – due to insulin secreted by hepatoma and fibrosarcoma.

Hematological paraneoplastic syndromes

- Erythrocytosis – seen in renal cell carcinoma, cerebellar hemangioblastoma and hepatocellular carcinoma
- Pure red cell aplasia – seen in thymomas
- Autoimmune hemolytic anemia – seen in B-cell neoplasms.
- Eosinophilia – seen in Hodgkin lymphoma
- Disseminated intravascular coagulation – seen in acute myeloid leukemia M3
- Venous thrombosis – seen in pancreatic carcinoma
- Non-bacterial thrombotic endocarditis – seen in leukemias and lymphomas.

PROTEIN ENERGY MALNUTRITION (PEM)

Definition: It is a spectrum of clinical features seen in young individuals due to deficient intake of proteins or calories or both way below bodily requirements.

Classification: (Based on etiology)

- Primary protein energy malnutrition
    - Kwashiorkor
    - Marasmus
- Secondary protein energy malnutrition
    - Kwashiorkor like syndrome
    - Marasmus like syndrome

Secondary protein energy malnutrition

- Causes
    - Acquired immunodeficiency syndrome (AIDS)
    - Cancers
    - Chronic gastrointestinal malabsorption
    - Old age
- Kwashiorkor like protein energy malnutrition seen in acute catabolic diseases, e.g. trauma, burns, sepsis and occurs in a period of few weeks
- Marasmus like illness seen in chronic lung diseases and develops in months.

Morphological features

- Growth retardation – seen in both kwashiorkor and marasmus
- Peripheral edema – seen more in kwashiorkor
- Loss of body fat and muscle atrophy – seen in marasmus
- Liver changes – seen more in kwashiorkor and comprise fatty liver
- Small intestinal changes – mucosal atrophy and loss of brush border
- Hematological changes – normocytic normochromic anemia is seen.

Marasmus

- It is a type of malnutrition due to severe reduction in calorie intake
- Somatic protein compartment is depleted
- Weight of child <60% of normal body weight
- There is loss of muscle and subcutaneous fat leading to emaciation of extremities
- Associated features:
    - Anemia
    - Multivitamin deficiency
    - T-cell immunodeficiency

Kwashiorkor

- It occurs due to more protein deprivation than calories
- More severe to marasmus
- It occurs due to depletion of visceral proteins causing hypoalbuminemia
- Weight of child is 60 – 80% of normal
- Somatic proteins are rarely affected
- Skin lesions – alternate areas of hyper and hypopigmentation giving flaky paint appearance
- Hair changes – loss of colour or alternate bands of pale and darker hairs
- Liver changes – steatosis is seen.

FAT SOLUBLE VITAMIN DISORDERS

Vitamin E deficiency disorder

- Causes
  - Malabsorption
  - Dietary deficiency
  - Premature infants
  - Abetalipoproteinemia patients
  - Genetic disorder of vitamin E metabolism
- Clinical features
  - Decrease or absent tendon reflexes
  - Dysarthria
  - Ataxia
  - Loss of position and vibration sense
  - Muscle weakness
  - Impaired vision
  - Ophthalmoplegia
  - High-risk of atherosclerosis.

Vitamin A deficiency disorder

- Causes
  - Inadequate intake
  - Malabsorption syndrome
- Clinical features
  - Impaired night vision due to decreased production of visual pigment
  - Eye changes – Bitot spots → corneal ulcer → keratomalacia → blindness
  - Squamous metaplasia of ducts causing dry eyes, follicular dermatitis and renal stones due to renal pelvic keratinization
  - Immunodeficiency.

Vitamin A excess disorder

- Acute vitamin A toxicity – characterized by:
  - Headache
  - Vomiting
  - Stupor
  - Papilledema
- Chronic vitamin A toxicity- characterized by:
  - Nausea and vomiting
  - Weight loss
  - Dryness of mucosa of lips
  - Orthodynia
  - Hyperostosis
  - Hepatic fibrosis

Vitamin K deficiency disorder

- Causes:
  - Malabsorption
  - Dietary deficiency
- Vitamin K deficiency causes decreased synthesis of clotting factor II, VII, IX and X
- Clinical features – Bleeding diathesis characterized by:
  - Hematomas
  - Purpura
  - Ecchymosis
  - Hematuria
  - Malena
  - Bleeding gums.

Vitamin D deficiency disorder

- It causes rickets in children and osteomalacia in adults
- Causes:
  - Dietary deficiency
  - Gastrointestinal malabsorption
  - Derangement in vitamin D metabolism
  - End organ resistance to vitamin D
- Clinical features – Skeletal deformities due to excess of unmineralized bone matrix
  - Craniotabes – Flattened occipital bone and elastic recoil in parietal bones
  - Frontal bossing of head
  - Rachitic rosary – due to thickening of costochondral junction
  - Pigeon breast deformity – Anterior protrusion of sternum
  - Harrison sulcus – Groove in ribcage due to pull of diaphragm
  - Excessive lumbar lordosis
  - Bowing of legs.

WATER SOLUBLE VITAMIN DISORDERS

Thiamine (Vitamin B_1) deficiency disorder

- Causes
  - Dietary deficiency
  - Chronic alcoholism
  - Pernicious vomiting of pregnancy
  - Malabsoption
- Clinical features – 3 distinct syndromes
  - Dry Beri-beri (Polyneuropathy)
    - Symmetric sensorimotor neuropathy
    - Foot drop
    - Wrist drop
    - Myasthenia
    - Hyporeflexia
  - Wet Beri-beri (Cardiovascular syndrome)
    - Peripheral vasodilation
    - High output cardiac failure
    - Peripheral edema
  - Wernicke's encephalopathy (WE) and Korsakoff psychosis (KP) syndrome
    - Ophthalmoplegia, Nystagmus, Ataxia, Confusion, Apathy, Listlessness } seen in WE
    - Retrograde amnesia, Confabulations } seen in KP

Riboflavin (Vitamin B_2) deficiency disorder

- Predisposing causes
  - Chronic alcoholism
  - Cancer cachexia
  - Anorexia nervosa
- Clinical features
  - Cheilosis
  - Glossitis
  - Superficial interstitial keratitis
  - Scaling dermatitis
  - Pure red cell aplasia
  - Skin atrophy.

Niacin (Vitamin B_5) deficiency

- Predisposing causes
  - Alcoholism
  - Chronic infections and illnesses
- Clinical features
  - Diarrhea
  - Dermatitis
  - Dementia

WATER SOLUBLE VITAMIN DISORDERS (contd.)

Vitamin C (Ascorbic acid) deficiency

- Predisposing causes
  - Dietary deficiency
  - Total peritoneal dialysis patients
  - Food faddist
  - Formula milk fed infants
- Clinical features
  - Skin hemorrhages
  - Purpura and ecchymoses
  - Subperiosteal hematoma
  - Hemarthrosis
  - Bleeding gums
  - Bone defects due to inadequate osteoid formation
  - Epiphyseal bone widening
  - Depression of sternum with protrusion of ribs
  - Scrobutic rosary – due to cartilage overgrowth of costochondral junction
  - Perifollicular hyperkeratotic papular rashes on skin
  - Impaired wound healing.

ACQUIRED IMMUNODEFICIENCY SYNDROME (AIDS)

Definition: It is defined as a disease caused by human immunodeficiency virus (HIV) and is characterized by immunosupression which leads to opportunistic infections and other manifestations.

Clinical manifestations

- HIV infection occurs in 3 phases:
  - *Early acute infection*
    - Occurs 3 – 6 weeks after infection
    - Non-specific clinical symptoms
    - Persistent generalized lymphadenopathy
    - CD4 + T-cell count > 500 cells/μL
  - *Middle chronic infection*
    - Occurs multiple years after infection
    - Symptoms due to impaired cell-mediated immunity
    - CD4 + T-cell count 200 – 499 cells/μL
  - *Final phase (progression to AIDS)*
    - Opportunistic infection develop
    - Neurodegenerative disease
    - Development of secondary malignancies
    - CD4 + T-cell count < 200 cells/μL.

Opportunisitc infections

- Cryptosporidiosis
- *Pneumocystic carinii* infection
- Toxoplasmosis
- Atypical mycobacterial infection
- Nocardiosis
- Esophageal or tracheal candidiasis
- Cryptococcal meningitis
- Coccidiomycosis
- Histoplasmosis
- *Cytomegalovirus* infection
- *Herpes simplex virus* infection
- *Varicella-Zoster virus* infection.

Opportunistic neoplasm

- Kaposi sarcoma
- B-cell non-Hodgkin lymphoma
- Central nervous system lymphoma
- Cervix carcinoma.

ACQUIRED IMMUNODEFICIENCY SYNDROME (AIDS) (contd.)

Pathogenesis

HIV virion is CD4 + T-cell tropic

↓

Glycoprotein 41 binds with CD4 receptor on T-cells

↓

Glycoprotein 120 enters into lipid membrane of CD4 + T-lymphocyte

↓

HIV RNA enters CD4 + T-cell cytoplasm

↓

HIV RNA converted to cDNA

↓

HIV DNA binds CD4 + T-cell nuclear DNA

↓

Activation of transcription factor NFκB

↓

Multiplication of viral DNA

↓

HIV DNA converted to HIV RNA

↓

Viral RNA released out of CD4 + T-cell

↓

Multiplication of HIV RNA destroys CD4 + T-cell by cytopathic effect, induction of apoptosis and by activation of CD8 + cytotoxic T-lymphocytes.

Etiology

- AIDS is caused by HIV, a retrovirus of lentivirus family
- HIV is of two types:
- HIV I – causes AIDS in USA, Europe and Africa
- HIV II – causes AIDS in India
- HIV contains following structures:
  - Core proteins p18 and p24
  - 2 strands of RNA
  - Reverse transcriptase enzyme
  - Outer double layered lipid membrane containing 2 envelop glycoproteins gp120 and gp41
- HIV infects humans by following routes:
  - Sexual contact (75% cases)
  - Parenteral transmission
  - Perinatal transmission
- High-risk groups
  - Homosexual men
  - Bisexual men
  - Intravenous drug abusers
  - Hemophiliacs
  - Blood transfusion recepeints
  - Healthcare workers.

TUBERCULOSIS

Definition: It is a chronic granulomatous infection caused by *Mycobacterium tuberculosis.*

Etiology

- Tuberculosis is caused by acid fast bacillus *Mycobacterium tuberculosis*
- Tuberculosis spreads by following routes:
  - Inhalation
  - Ingestion
  - Inoculation
  - Transplacental route
- Tuberculosis spreads in human body by:
  - Local spread
  - Lymphatic spread
  - Hematogenous spread
  - Body cavity spread
- High-risk individuals:
  - Diabetes mellitus patients
  - AIDS patients
  - Hodgkin lymphoma patients
  - Chronic renal failure patients
  - Malnutrition
  - Alcoholics
  - Immunosupressed individuals.

Complications

- Fibrosis
- Pulmonary insufficiency
- Pulmonary hemorrhage
- Sepsis
- Corpulmonale
- Amyloidosis

Pathogenesis

- M. tuberculosis infects macrophages
- This antigen presenting cell induces type IV hypersensitivity reaction which leads to formation of granulomas associated with caseous necrosis.

TUBERCULOSIS (contd.)

Morphology

Microscopy (Fig. 4)

- Formation of caseating and noncaseating granulomas
- Granulomas are surrounded by lymphocytes, fibroblasts and collagen
- Granulomas are composed of epithelioid histiocytes and multinucleated Langhans type of giant cells.

Gross morphology

- *Primary tuberculosis* **(Image G)**
  - The bacilli implant in lower part of upper lobe and upper part of lower lobe of lung
  - 1–1.5 cm grey white focus of consolidation called Ghon focus
  - Ghon focus with hilar lymph node and lymphatics is called Ghon complex
  - Ghon complex undergo calcification to form Ranke complex
- *Secondary tuberculosis* **(Image H)**
  - 1–2 cm lesion in apex of lung
  - Lesion is well-circumscribed, grey white with central caseation and peripheral fibrosis
- *Progressive pulmonary tuberculosis*
  - In this, the lesion open into airspace releasing necrotic material
  - There is formation of fibrocaseous cavity
- *Miliary tuberculosis* **(Image I)**
  - Multiple lesions formed in lung measuring 1–2 mm throughout its parenchyma due to hematogenous spread.

ANEMIA

Definition: It is defined as a decrease in competence of blood to carry oxygen to tissues leading to tissue hypoxia due to decease in concentration of hemoglobin or erythrocytes.

Lab investigations

- Erythrocyte count
- Hematocrit
- Hemoglobin
- Erythrocyte indices – mean corpuscular volume (MCV), mean corpuscular hemoglobin (MCH), mean corpuscular hemoglobin concentration (MCHC)
- Peripheral blood smear examination
- Reticulocyte count
- Leukocyte and platelet quantitative and qualitative examination
- Bone marrow examination
- Tests for erythrocyte destruction – serum bilirubin, serum haptoglobin, urine hemosiderin, serum lactate dehydrogenase.

Classification

Morphological classification (Based on average size and hemoglobin concentration)

Microcytic hypochromic anemia

- Iron deficiency anemia **(Fig. 22)**
- Thalassemia **(Fig. 23)**
- Anemia of chronic disease
- Sideroblastic anemia
- Hemoglobinopathies
- Lead toxicity
- Porphyrias.

Macrocytic normochronic anemia

- Vitamin B_{12} and folic acid deficiency **(Fig. 25)**
- Myelodysplastic syndromes
- Liver disease
- Alcoholism
- Drug induced macrocytosis.

Normocytic normochromic anemia

- Aplastic anemia
- Pure red cell aplasia
- Immune hemolytic anemia **(Fig. 26)**
- Acute hemorrhage

ANEMIA (contd.) → **Classification (contd.)** → **Functional classification**

Increased red cell destruction
- Intrinsic (intracorpuscular) defect
  - Hereditary elliptocytosis
  - Glucose-6-phosphate dehydrogenase deficiency
  - Pyruvate kinase deficiency
  - Thalassemia
  - Sickle cell anemia
  - Paroxysmal nocturnal hemoglobinuria
- Extrinsic (extracorpuscular) defect
  - Autoimmune hemolytic anemia
  - Transfusion reaction
  - Thrombotic thrombocytopenic purpura
  - Disseminated intravascular coagulation
  - Malaria
  - Hookworm infection
  - Lead poisoning.

Impaired erythrocyte production
- Aplastic anemia
- Pure red cell aplasia
- Anemia of renal failure
- Vitamin B_{12} and folate deficiency anemia
- Iron deficiency anemia
- Thalassemia
- Sideroblastic anemia
- Anemia of chronic disease
- Myelophthisic anemia.

Blood loss anemia
- Trauma
- Menorrhagia
- Gastrointestinal bleeding

IRON DEFICIENCY ANEMIA

Definition: It is the most common type of nutritional anemia in world caused by deficiency of iron in human body.

Clinical features

- Insidious onset
- Weakness
- Fatigue
- Lethargy
- Pica (perversion of apetite leading to bizarre eating practices)
- Irritability
- Memory loss
- Deficient learning.

Etiology: Causes of iron deficiency include:

- Blood loss
  - Peptic ulcer
  - Gastric malignancies
  - Alcoholic gastritis
  - Salicylate ingestion
  - Hookworm infection
  - Hemorrhoids
- Inadequate dietary intake
  - Infants
  - Pregnancy
  - Adolescents
  - Poor diet due to low socioeconomic status
  - Malabsorption
  - Tropical sprue
  - Post-gastrectomy
  - Atrophic gastritis
  - Achlorhydria.

Laboratory investigations

Peripheral blood smear finding (Fig. 22)

- Deceased hemoglobin (Mean Hb–8.4 g%)
- Decreased MCV (55–74 fl)
- Decreased MCH (14–26 pg)
- Decreased MCHC (22–31 g/dl)
- Increased red cell distribution width (RDW)
- Erythrocytes are microcytic and hypochromic with few target cells and elliptocytes
- Leucocytes are normal or increased with eosinophilia in hookworm infestation
- Platelets are normal, increased or decreased
- Reticulocyte percentage is reduced.

Bone marrow findings

- Micronormoblastic erythroid hyperplasia

Other investigations

- Iron studies:
  - Serum iron–decreased (<30 mg/dl)
  - Total iron binding capacity – increased
  - Transferrin saturation decreased (<15%)
  - Serum ferritin – decreased (<12 mg/L)

THALASSEMIA

Definition: It is a heterogenous group of inherited disorders caused by genetic mutation in α or β globin genes leading to deficient production of α and β-globin chains of hemoglobin A.

Pathogenesis

- Hemoglobin A is composed of 2α and 2β globin chains coded by two α globin genes on chromosome 16 and one β-globin gene on chromosome 11
- β-thalassemia occurs due to mutations in β-globin gene leading to deficient or absent β-globin protein synthesis
- α-thalassemia occurs due to mutation in α-globin gene leading to impaired synthesis of α-globin protein.

Clinical features

- Symptoms of anemia
- Failure to thrive and gain weight
- Diarrhea, fever and enlarged abdomen
- Growth retardation; brown pigmentation of skin
- Massive splenomegaly
- Facial bone deformities with frontal bossing of skull with hair on end appearance on X-ray
- Gallstones, gout and icterus due to hemolysis.

Laboratory investigations

Peripheral blood smear findings (Fig. 23)

- Hemoglobin – low; 2 – 3 g/dl in thalassemia major
- MCV – decreased
- MCH – decreased
- MCHC – decreased
- Erythrocytes are microcytic and hypochromic with schistocytes, ovalocytes, target cells, polychromatophilic and nucleated erythrocytes seen
- Leucocytes and thrombocytes are normal
- RDW – increased
- Reticulocyte count – increased (<10%)

Bone marrow findings

- Micronormoblastic erythroid hyperplasia with Myeloid: Erythroid ratio of upto 1: 10.

Other investigations

- Iron studies –
  - Serum iron – normal or increased
  - Total iron binding capacity – normal or decreased
  - Transferrin saturation – increased
  - Serum ferritin – normal or increased
- Hemoglobin electrophoresis – in thalassemia major, absence of HbA with 90% HbF and low, normal or increased HbA2.

Classification

Classification of α-thalassemia

- Hydrops fetalis – No α-chain synthesis; lethal *in utero*
- Hemoglobin H disease – Severe anemia resembling thalassemia intermedia.
- α-thalassemia trait – Asymptomatic resembling thalassemia minor
- Sillent carrier – No erythrocyte abnormality.

Classification of β-thalassemia

- Thalassemia major – Severe anemia occurs which requires blood transfusion
- Thalassemia intermedia – Severe disease which does not require blood transfusion
- Thalassemia minor – Asymptomatic with mild or no anemia.

SICKLE CELL ANEMIA

Definition: It is a type of hereditary hemoglobinopathy characterized by production of defective hemoglobin (HbS).

Etiopathogenesis

- Hemoglobin is formed due to point mutation at sixth position of β-globin chain leading to substitution of valine for glutamic acid
- Under deoxygenated state, HbS is aggregated and polymerized converting liquid cell cytosol to viscid gel
- On oxygenation, it depolymerizes but repeated deoxygenation makes it an irreversible process
- Irreversibly sickled cells are destroyed in spleen.

Clinical features

- Symptoms appear at 6 months of age
- Symptoms of moderate to severe chronic hemolytic anemia
- Vasoocclusive crisis – due to blockade of microvasculature leading to infarction of genitourinary tract, liver bone, lung and spleen; dactylitis with chronic leg ulcers.
- Spleen is enlarged first followed by infarction and fibrosis leading to autosplenectomy by 10 years of age
- Bacterial infection like pneumonia is commonly seen
- Aplastic crisis – After early erythroid hyperplasia, the bone marrow undergo hypoplasia followed by aplasia leading to infections and bleeding manifestations.

Laboratory investigations

Peripheral blood smear findings (Fig. 24)

- Hemoglobin – decreased (6–10 g%)
- Hematocrit – 18–30%
- Reticulocyte count – increased (10–20%)
- Erythrocytes are normocytic and normochromic with presence of sickled cells and target cells
- Leucocytes are normal or decreased
- Platelets are normal, increased or decreased
- RDW – Increased

Other investigations

- Hemoglobin electrophoresis – At pH 8.5 on cellulose acetate, 85 – 90% HbS is detected with rest being HbF and HbA_2; HbA is absent
- Sickling test – Blood is deoxygenated with sodium metabisulphite and examined under the microscope on a glass slide with sealed coverslip after 30 minutes show sickle cells.

Bone marrow findings

- Marrow shows erythroid hyperplasia

HEREDITARY SPHEROCYTOSIS (HS)

Definition: It is an inherited disorder caused by intrinsic defects in erythrocyte cell membrane that transforms normal discoid erythrocytes into spherocytes leading to their splenic sequestration and destruction.

Etiopathogenesis
- Disease is predominantly autosomal dominant; rarely autosomal recessive
- The erythrocyte membrane defect is characterized by a primary deficiency of spectrin or secondary deficiency due to defective attachment of skeleton to lipid bilayer.
- Dyscoordination between skeletal proteins and lipid bilayer leads to loss of lipid bilayer changing the morphology from discocyte to spherocyte
- Less deformability of spherocytes leads to splenic sequestration and its destruction.

Clinical features
- Symptoms appear in infancy or childhood
- Symptoms of mild to moderate anemia
- Intermittent jaundice
- Splenomegaly
- Cholelithiasis in late stages
- Aplastic crisis – Develops after acute parvovirus infection.

Laboratory investigations

Peripheral blood smear findings (Fig. 24)
- Hemoglobin – decreased (8–11 g%) in infants; older children have >10 g%
- MCV—decreased or normal
- MCH—normal
- MCHC—increased; spherocytes are the only type of erythrocytes with increased MCHC
- Reticulocyte count—increased (>8%)
- Erythrocytes are normocytic, normochromic or microcytic, hypochromic with presence of spherocytes
- Leucocytes are normal or decreased
- Platelets are normal, increased or decreased

Other investigations
- Osmotic fragility test: It is the confirmatory test for HS; normal erythrocytes hemolysis start and complete at 0.5% and 0.3% NaCl solution respectively; hemolysis of spherocytes of HS start and complete at 0.7% and 0.4% NaCl solution.

Bone marrow findings
- Marrow shows normoblastic erythroid hyperplasia

MACROCYTIC ANEMIA

Definition: It is a type of anemia characterized by large erythrocytes with mean corpuscular volume >100 fL that have a normal hemoglobin content in relation to their size.

Clinical features

- Symptoms of anemia, i.e. lethargy, weakness and pallor
- Dyspepsia
- Glossitis with beefy red tongue
- Loss of weight and apetite
- Diarrhea
- Neurological symptoms, i.e. tingling, numbness, weakness of extremities, loss of vibration and proprioception, loss of memory, depression and irritability are seen in vitamin B_{12} deficiency anemia.

Classification: It is classified into 2 groups:

- *Megaloblastic macrocytic anemia*: In this type, megaloblasts are seen which are erythroid precursors seen in bone marrow due to abnormal DNA synthesis
  - Vitamin B_{12} deficiency
  - Folic acid deficiency
  - Myelodysplastic syndromes
  - Chemotherapy effects
- *Non-megaloblastic macrocytic anemia*: In this type, there are no megaloblasts seen in bone marrow
  - Alcoholism
  - Liver disease
  - Hemolysis
  - Hypothyroidism.

Laboratory investigations

Peripheral blood findings (Fig. 25)

- Macrocytic normochromic anemia with triad of macrovalocytes, Howell-Jolly bodies and hypersgmented neutrophils
- Red cell indices
  - MCV >100 fL
  - MCH >33pg
  - MCHC is normal
- Hemoglobin – Normal to very low
- RBC count – Normal to very low
- WBC count – Normal to decreased
- Platelet count – Normal to decreased.

Bone marrow findings

- Bone marrow shows erythroid hyperplasia with presence of megaloblasts
- Megaloblasts are large nucleated erythroid precursor in which nuclear maturation lags behind cytoplasmic maturation
- Megaloblasts show bluish grey cytoplasm and nucleus with loose open chromatin
- Giant metamyelocytes and myelocytes with poor granulation seen
- Megakaryocytes are normal, increased or decreased.

Other lab findings

- Serum lactate dehydrogenase levels are elevated
- Increased forminoglutamic acid (FIGLU) in urine after histidine administration
- Serum haptoglobin, uric acid and alkaline phosphatase are decreased
- Serum and erythrocyte cobalamine levels are decreased in vitamin B_{12} deficiency anemia
- Serum and erythrocytes folate levels are decreased in folate deficiency anemia
- Schilling test – It is a definitive test useful in distinguishing vitamin B_{12} deficiency due to malabsorption, dietary deficiency or absence of intrinsic factor.

APLASTIC ANEMIA

Clinical features
- Bleeding with skin hemorrhages
- Symptoms of anemia
- Infections leading to fever.

Definition: It is a pluripotent stem cell disorder characterized by peripheral pancytopenia and accompanied by a hypocellular bone marrow.

Etiology: Causes of aplastic anemia are:
- *Acquired causes*
  - Idiopathic
  - Drugs – Chloramphenicol, phenylbutazone, gold, sulfa drugs, antihistamines, phenytoin
  - Chemicals – Benzene, insecticides, hair dyes, carbon tetrachloride, arsenic, cancer chemotherapeutic agents like vincristine and busulfan
  - Ionizing radiations
  - Infections – Human parvovirus, infectious mononucleosus, hepatitis, measles and influenza
  - Pregnancy
  - Paroxymal nocturnal hemoglobinuria
- *Congenital causes*
  - Fanconi anemia
  - Familial aplastic anemia
  - Diamond Blackfan syndrome.

Laboratory investigations

Peripheral blood findings
- Hemoglobin <7 g%
- Erythrocytes are reduced in number with normocytic and normochromic appearance.
- Leukocytes are reduced in number; neutropenia preceeds leucopenia; lymphocytes and monocyte counts are normal.
- Platelets are reduced in number.

Bone marrow findings
- Bone marrow is hypocellular with >70% fat
- Bone marrow aspiration is different and often yields dry tap.

HEMOLYTIC ANEMIA

Definition: They are a heterogeneous group of normocytic normochromic anemias in which erythrocytes are prematurely destroyed intravascularly in circulation or extravascularly in spleen.

Hemolytic anemias with extravascular hemolysis

- *Intreited erythrocyte defects*
  - Thalassemia
  - Hemoglobinopathies
  - Enzyme deficiencies
  - Membrane disorders
- *Acquired erythrocyte defects*
  - Megaloblastic anemia
  - Spur cell anemia
- *Immune hemolytic anemias*
  - Autoimmune
  - Drug induced.

Classification

- Intrinsic (inherited)
  - Membrane defects
    - Hereditary spherocytosis
    - Hereditary elliptocytosis
    - Hereditary xerocytosis
    - Paroxysmal nocturnal hemoglobinuria
  - Enzyme deficiency
    - G-6-PD deficiency
    - Pyruvate kinase deficiency
  - Abnormal hemoglobin
    - Thalassemia
    - Structural hemoglobin variants
- Extrinsic (acquired)
  - Antagonistic plasma factors
    - Chemicals
    - Drugs
    - Insect venom
    - Infections
  - Traumatic injury
  - Immune mediated cell destruction
    - Autoimmune hemolytic anemia (AIHA)
    - Alloimmune hemolytic anemia
    - Drug induced.

Laboratory investigations

Lab findings reflecting increased erythrocyte destruction (Fig. 26)

- Anemia
- Poikilocytes such as spherocytes and schistocytes
- Decreased serum haptoglobin
- Decreased glycosylated hemoglobin
- Increased serum unconjugated bilirubin
- Increased fecal and urine urobilinogen
- Positive Coomb test (in AIHA)
- Hemoglobinemia, hemoglobinuria, hemosiderinuria and methemoglobinemia seen in intravascular hemolytic anemias.

Lab findings reflecting increased bone marrow activity

- Reticulocytosis
- Leucocytosis
- Nucleated erythrocytes in peripheral blood
- Polychromasia of erythrocytes
- Normoblastic erythroid hyperplasia in bone marrow.

Definition: They are a group of disorders characterized by panhypercellularity of bone marrow accompanied by erythrocytosis, granulocytosis and thrombocytosis in the peripheral blood.

Pathophysiology

- There is increased number of pluripotent stem cells which are abnormal.
- There are abnormal pluripotent stem cells proliferate along one cell line under the influence of various growth factors –
  - Plasma PDGF levels are increased in myelofibrosis and essential thrombocythemia
  - Serum colony stimulating factor 1 levels are elevated in all MPD
  - The increase in growth factors occur due to overexpression of proto-oncogenes caused by mutations.

CHRONIC MYELOPROLIFERATIVE DISORDERS (MPDs)

Classification (Based on predominant cell line involved)

- **Mast cells** → **Systemic mastocytosis**
- **Fibroblast** → **Myelofibrosis with myeloid metaplasia**
- **Erythroid** → **Polycythemia rubra vera**
- **Myeloid** → **Chronic eosinophilic leukemia**; **Chronic myeloid leukemia**; **Chronic neutrophilic leukemia**
- **Megakaryocytic** → **Essential Thrombocythemia**

CHRONIC MYELOID LEUKEMIA

Definition: It is the most common MPD characterized by neoplastic growth of primary myeloid cells in the bone marrow with extreme elevation of these cells in peripheral blood.

Pathophysiology

- A chromosomal abnormality, i.e. Philadelphia chromosome is seen in all hematopoietic cells in 90–95% patients
- Philadelphia chromosome is formed by reciprocal translocation of ABL gene on chromosome 9q34 to BCR gene on chromosome 22q11.
- ABL–BCR gene gives rise to an abnormal protein which has tyrosine kinase like activity leading to uncontrolled proliferation of myeloid cells.

Clinical features

- Age group–Middle age, peak in 40–50 years
- Sex – M : F : : 1 : 1
- Insidious onset with constitutional symptoms like weakness, fever, sweats, weightloss and fullness of abdomen
- Examination findings – Pallor, retinal hemorrhages, petechiae and ecchymoses, sternal tenderness and splenomegaly.

Blast crisis phase

- It occurs 30–40 months after diagnosis
- Clinically, patients debilitation increases with pyrexia, night sweats, weightloss, weakness, malaise, bone pain with splenomegaly and refractoriness to chemotherapy
- Laboratory investigations reveal worsening of anemia, thrombocytopenia, increased basophilia and increase in myeloblasts in peripheral blood and bone marrow (>20%).

CHRONIC MYELOID LEUKEMIA (contd.)

Laboratory investigations

Peripheral blood findings (Fig. 27)

- Normocytic normochromic anemia with occasional nucleated erythrocytes
- Leucocytosis (100 – 500 × $10^3/\mu L$)
- Shift to left of myeloid series with predominance of myelocytes and neutrophils
- Monocytosis
- Basophilia
- Eosinophilia
- Neutrophils show decreased nuclear lobes (Pseudo Pelger Heut anomaly)

Bone marrow finding

- Bone marrow is hypercellular with myeloid to erythroid ratio between 10 : 1 to 50 : 1
- There are primary granulocytic precursors seen with <20% myeloblasts
- Erythropoeisis is normoblastic
- Megakaryocytes are increased in number with immature and atypical forms
- Pseudo Gaucher cells are seen admixed with hematopoietic elements
- In late stages, bone marrow fibrosis ensues.

Other findings

- Decreased leucocyte alkaline phosphatase levels
- Serum total cobalamine levels are increased
- Serum uric acid and lactate dehydrogenase levels are elevated.

POLYCYTHEMIA RUBRA VERA

Definition: It is a myeloproliferative disorder characterized by unregulated proliferation of erythroid elements in the bone marrow and an increase in erythrocyte concentration in peripheral blood.

Classification
- Polycythemia vera
- Secondary polycythemia
  - Appropriate erythropoietin production
    - High attitude
    - Chronic obstructive pulmonary disease
    - Pickwickian syndrome
  - Inappropriate erythropoietin production
    - Tumor
    - Renal ischemia
- Familial erythrocytosis.

Pathophysiology
- It is a clonal stem cell defect in which proliferation of erythroid series of cells occur probably due to following mechanisms:
- Erythropoeitin independent proliferation of neoplastic stem cells
- Hypersensitivity of erythroid stem cells to erythropoietin
- Hypersensitivity of erythroid stem cells to growth factors other than erythropoietin
- Presence of abnormal growth factors acting on normal stem cells.

Clinical features
- Age group: 40–60 years; peak in sixth decade of life
- Sex: Males are affected more than females
- Headache, weakness, pruritis, weight loss and fatigue due to increased erythrocyte mass
- Gingival bleeding, menorrhagia, hemoptysis, gastrointestinal bleeding
- Splenomgaly and hepatomegaly
- In late stages; anemia symptoms, infection and bleeding occur due to bone marrow failure.

Laboratory investigations

Other laboratory findings
- Serum uric acid >7 mg/dl
- Serum cobalamin levels are elevated.

Peripheral blood findings
- Hemoglobin >18g%
- Hematocrit: 55–60 L/L
- Erythrocyte count: $6–10 \times 10^6/\mu l$
- Erythrocytes are normocytic and normochromic in early stages with microcytic and hypochromic cells in late stages due to iron deficiency
- Leucocyte count is $12–20 \times 10^3/\mu l$ with mild shift to left
- Platelets count $>400 \times 10^3/\mu l$.

Bone marrow findings
- Moderate to marked increase in bone marrow cellularity
- Myeloid to erythroid ratio is normal
- Eosinophilic precursors are increased
- Megakaryocytes are increased in number.

ACUTE MYELOID LEUKEMIA (AML)

Definition: It is a stem cell disorder characterized by a malignant neoplastic proliferation and accumulation of immature myeloid cells in the bone marrow.

Clinical features

- Symptoms of anemia
- Bleeding, bruising and petechial hemorrhages due to thrombocytopenia
- Bone tenderness, hepatosplenomegaly and lymphadenopathy in 50% patients
- Patients with AML M3 develop DIC.

Classification (based on FAB classification system) AML is classified into 8 subclasses:

- Minimally differentiated AML (M_0)
- AML without differentiation (M_1)
- AML with maturation (M_2)
- Acute promyelocytic leukemia (M_3)
- Acute myelomonocytic leukemia (M_4)
- Acute monocytic leukemia (M_5)
- Acute erythroleukemia (M_6)
- Acute megakaryocytic leukemia (M_7).

Laboratory investigations

Peripheral blood findings (Fig. 28)

- Normocytic normochromic anemia with nucleated erythrocytes
- Mild thrombocytopenia with few giant and hypogranular forms
- Leukocytes are increased in number with 20–95% myeloblasts
- Myeloblasts may contain Auer rods (seen in M1, M2, M3)
- Monocytosis, eosinophilia and basophilia may be noted
- Neutropenia with hypolobated and hypogranular neutrophils.

Other laboratory findings

- Serum uric acid >7 mg/dl
- Increased serum lactate dehydrogenase
- Serum and urine muramidase elevated in M4 and M5 AML
- PT and APTT are prolonged in AML

Bone marrow findings

- Bone marrow is hypercellular with >20% myeloblasts
- Myeloblasts stain positive for myeloperoxidase and Sudan black B stain
- Dysplasia of leukocytes, erythrocytes and hypolobation of megakaryocytes may be seen.

ACUTE LYMPHOBLASTIC LEUKEMIA (ALL)

Definition: It is a stem cell disorder characterized by malignant neoplastic proliferation and accumulation of immature lymphoid cells is bone marrow and other organs.

Clinical findings

- Age group – Young children; peak in Ist decade
- Symptoms of anemia
- Symptoms of neutropenia
- Symptoms of thrombocytopenia
- Bone pain and sternal tenderness in 80% patients
- Headache and vomiting secondary to central nervous system involvement
- Hepatosplenomegaly and lymphadenopathy are commonly seen.

Laboratory investigations

Bone marrow findings

- Bone marrow is hypercellular with lymphoblasts comprising >30% of all nucleated cells
- Lymphoblasts stain positive for Periodic acid Schiff (PAS) and terminal deoxynucleotidyl transferase (TdT) stain and are negative for myeloperoxidase and Sudan black B stains.

Peripheral blood findings (Fig. 29)

- Normocytic normochromic anemia
- Leucocyte count is increased, normal or decreased with marked neutropenia
- Lymphoblasts >20% of all leukocytes are seen and have scant cytoplasm, large nucleus with indistinct chromatin and absent nucleoli
- Thrombocytopenia.

Classification (FAB classification based on lymphoblast morphology)

L_1 ALL

- Most common in children
- Best prognosis
- Lymphoblasts are small (twice the size of small lymphocytes) with scant basophilic cytoplasm and regular nucleus with occasional clefts, homogenous chromatin and absence of nucleoli.

L_2 ALL

- Most common in adults
- Lymphoblasts are large with abundant basophilic cytoplasm containing fine granules and irregular nucleus with indentations, heterogeneous chromatin and variable number of nucleoli.

L_3 ALL (Burkitt Type)

- Rare; seen in children as well as adults
- Lymphoblasts are large with abundant vacuolated basophilic cytoplasm and oval to round nucleus with finely stippled chromatin and one or more nucleoli.

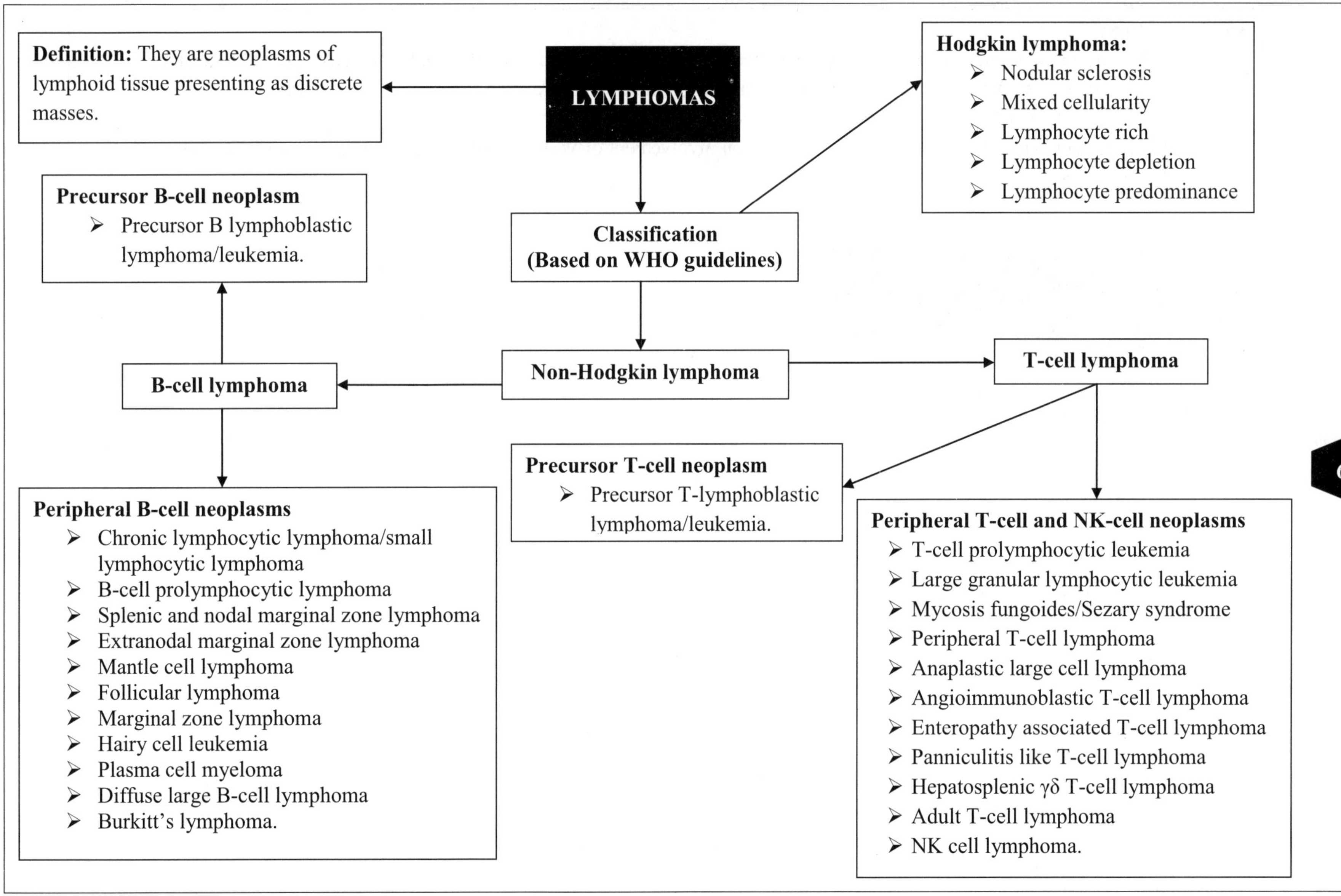
LYMPHOMAS
Definition: They are neoplasms of lymphoid tissue presenting as discrete masses.
Classification (Based on WHO guidelines)
Hodgkin lymphoma:
➢ Nodular sclerosis
➢ Mixed cellularity
➢ Lymphocyte rich
➢ Lymphocyte depletion
➢ Lymphocyte predominance
Non-Hodgkin lymphoma
B-cell lymphoma
T-cell lymphoma
Precursor B-cell neoplasm
➢ Precursor B lymphoblastic lymphoma/leukemia.
Peripheral B-cell neoplasms
➢ Chronic lymphocytic lymphoma/small lymphocytic lymphoma
➢ B-cell prolymphocytic lymphoma
➢ Splenic and nodal marginal zone lymphoma
➢ Extranodal marginal zone lymphoma
➢ Mantle cell lymphoma
➢ Follicular lymphoma
➢ Marginal zone lymphoma
➢ Hairy cell leukemia
➢ Plasma cell myeloma
➢ Diffuse large B-cell lymphoma
➢ Burkitt's lymphoma.
Precursor T-cell neoplasm
➢ Precursor T-lymphoblastic lymphoma/leukemia.
Peripheral T-cell and NK-cell neoplasms
➢ T-cell prolymphocytic leukemia
➢ Large granular lymphocytic leukemia
➢ Mycosis fungoides/Sezary syndrome
➢ Peripheral T-cell lymphoma
➢ Anaplastic large cell lymphoma
➢ Angioimmunoblastic T-cell lymphoma
➢ Enteropathy associated T-cell lymphoma
➢ Panniculitis like T-cell lymphoma
➢ Hepatosplenic γδ T-cell lymphoma
➢ Adult T-cell lymphoma
➢ NK cell lymphoma.

Specific features

- 80–90% of lymphoid neoplasms are B-cell lymphomas whereas T-cell and NK cell lymphoma constitute the remainder
- Lymphomas cause alteration in structure and function of immune system leading to immune abnormalitites
- NHL frequently involve multiple group of lymph nodes
- NHL spread in non-contiguous manner with common involvement of Waldeyer ring and mesenteric group of lymph nodes
- NHL often shows involvement of extranodal sites.

NON-HODGKIN LYMPHOMA (NHL)

Burkitt lymphoma

- It comprise 30% of all NHL
- Age – Children and young adults
- Types:
  - African (Endemic) Burkitt's lymphoma – It is associated with Epstein- Barr virus involvement
  - Sporadic Burkitt's lymphoma – It is more agressive than African type
  - HIV associated Burkitt's lymphoma
- It presents more often extranodally as compared to lymph nodes
- Morphology:
  - Diffuse effacement of lymph node by tumor cells 16 – 24 cm in diameter having moderate basophilic cytoplasm and round to oval nuclei with coarse chromatin and multiple nucleoli
  - Mitotic activity is high
  - Presence of benign macrophages in between leads to starry sky appearance under low power microscope
- Immunophenotype – Tumor cells are CD19, CD20 and CD10 positive
- Cytogenetics – translocation t (8; 14); t (2; 8) and t (2; 22) seen.

NON-HODGKIN LYMPHOMA (NHL) (contd.)

Follicular lymphoma

- It is the most common type of adult NHL
- It comprise 40–50% of all NHL
- Age – Middle adult; M : F : : 1 : 1
- Morphology–
  - Nodular or diffuse involvement of lymph node
  - 2 types of cells seen:
    - Centrocytes (Small cleaved cells) with scant cytoplasm and irregular nuclear contours
    - Centroblasts with moderate cytoplasm and nucleus showing open chromatin and multiple nucleoli
  - Immunophenotype – Tumor cells are CD19, 20, CD10 and CD25 positive but CD5 is negative.
  - Cytogenetics – Translocation t (14; 18) is seen in 90% cases.

Chronic lymphocytic leukemia (CLL)/small lymphocytic lymphoma (SLL) (Fig. 30)

- It constitutes 4% of all NHL
- Age – 50 – 70 years; M : F : : 2 : 1
- Clinical features–Fever, fatigue, weightloss, anorexia, lymphadenopathy, hepatosplenomegaly
- Richter syndrome – It is transformation of SLL to diffuse large B-cell lymphoma and occurs in 10% patients
- Morphology:
  - There is diffuse effacement of lymph node by small lymphocytes measuring 6 – 12 μm with scanty cytoplasm and round to irregular nuclei
  - There are prolymphocytes seen in between
  - Peripheral blood shows small lymphocyte lymphocytosis
- Immunophenotype – SLL tumor cells are CD19, CD20 as well as CD5 and CD23 positive.

HODGKIN LYMPHOMA (HL)

Specific features

- It accounts for 8% of all lymphoid neoplasms
- Most distinctive features are in presence of Reed-Sternberg (R-S) cell
- Peak incidence is seen between 15–55 years and beyond 50 years of age
- It is often localized to single group of lymph nodes and spread orderly to adjacent groups of lymph nodes
- Extra nodal involvement is rare in Hodgkin lymphoma
- Mesenteric nodes and waldeyer ring are rarely involved in Hodgkin lymphoma.

Morphology

Microscopy (Fig. 31)

- Diagnostic cell seen is Reed-Sternberg cell, 15–45 µm in diameter with multiple nuclei having large 5–7 µm nucleolus and abundant cytoplasm
- Variable amounts of plasma cells, macrophages eosinophils and fibrosis noted
- R-S cells are CD15 and CD30 positive.

Gross morphology

- Lymph nodes are enlarged and matted
- Cut surface shows fish flesh appearance.

Classification (Based on WHO guidelines)

Lymphocyte rich Hodgkin lymphoma

- It has the best prognosis amongst all subtypes of Hodgkin lymphoma
- Epstein-Barr virus is associated in 40% cases
- Lymphocytes form predominant cell infiltrate
- Classical R-S cells and Hodgkin cells are seen.

Mixed cellularity HL

- It comprises 20–25% cases of HL
- Epstein-Barr virus is associated in majority of cases
- Hodgkin cells (Mononuclear variant of Reed-Sternberg cell) are seen along with classical R-S cells.

Lymphocyte depletion HL

- It comprise <5% of all cases of HL
- It is commonly seen in elderly and HIV positive individual and has worst prognosis amongst all subtypes of HL
- Epstein-Barr virus association is commonly seen
- Classic R-S cells with very few small T-lymphocytes seen.

Nodular sclerosis HL

- It is the most common type of HL seen in 60–75% cases
- Lacunar cells – a variant of R-S cell which has multilobated nucleus and abundant cytoplasm disrupted during microtomy which makes the nuclei sitting in a lacuna
- Fibrosis varies from scanty to abundant
- There is no Epstein-Barr virus associated noted.

Lymphocyte predominance HL

- It accounts for 5% cases
- Popcorn cell (L and H cell) having delicate multilobated nucleus are seen
- There is lack of classical R-S cells, eosinophils, plasma cells and fibrosis
- The R-S cells in this subtype are CD30 and CD15 negative contrary to other subtypes
- Epstein-Barr virus has no association with it.

MULTIPLE MYELOMA

Definition: It is a neoplastic plasma cell dyscrasia characterized by a clinical pentad of anemia, monoclonal proteins in serum, urine or both, abnormal bone radiograph, hypercalcemia and renal insufficiency.

Etiopathogenesis

- Mutations are induced in cell regulator genes due to variable etiological factors including radiation exposure, viral infections etc.
- There is overexpression of cyclin D1 gene due to translocation between 11 and 14 chromosomes.
- This mutation causes unregulated proliferation of plasma cells.

Clinical features

- Recurrent infections
- Symptoms of anemia
- Easy bruisability
- Bone pain
- Symptoms of hypercalcemia
- Lytic bone lesions
- Hyperviscosity leading to thrombotic tendencies.

Laboratory investigations

Peripheral blood findings

- Haemoglobin <12 gm %
- Normocytic normochromic anemia with increased rouleaux formation
- Total leucocyte count and platelets are reduced in number.

Bone marrow findings (Fig. 32)

- Hypercellular marrow with >30% plasma cells comprising nonerythroid cells
- Erythroid and myeloid series are reduced in number.

Other laboratory findings

- Urinary Bence Jones proteins – These proteins have special feature that they coagulate on heating at 60–70°C but disappear on heating upto 100°C; On cooling they reappeared at 60°C
- Serum electrophoresis – M band composed of light chains of immunoglobulins is seen which is IgG in majority of cases
- Serum calcium levels – Elevated (>11 mg/dl)
- Serum creatinine >2 mg/dl is noted due to renal insufficiency.

IMMUNE THROMBOCYTOPENIC PURPURA (ITP)

Definition: It is a disorder characterized by decrease in platelet counts secondary to autoimmune destruction.

Etiopathogenesis
- Autoimmune destruction of platelets occurs by type II hypersensitivity
- Autoantibodies are formed against glycoprotein IIb/IIIa and Ib/IX on platelet surface
- Splenic macrophages recognize these antibodies by their Fc receptor and destroy them leading to destruction of platelets.

Classification (Based on duration)

Acute ITP
- It is seen in children between 2–6 years of age
- It follows viral infection by 1–3 weeks
- There is abrupt onset of bleeding in skin and mucous membranes
- Male : female ratio is 1 : 1
- Platelet count is usually <20,000/µl associated with eosinophilia and lymphocytosis
- The symptoms last for 2–6 weeks with spontaneous remission in 80% cases.

Chronic ITP
- It is seen in adults between 20–40 years of age
- Onset of bleeding is insidious without any antecedent cause
- Female : Male ratio is 3 : 1
- Platelet counts are usually between 30,000–80,000/µl
- Eosinophilia and lymphocytosis are rare
- The symptoms last for months to years with rare spontaneous remission
- Corticosteroids and splenectomy required for treatment.

Laboratory investigations

Peripheral blood findings
- Thrombocytopenia with presence of giant platelets are only significant finding
- Eosinophilia and lymphocytosis may be noted in acute ITP but is rare in chronic ITP.

Other findings
- Serum level of immunoglobulin G antibody against platelet surface glycoprotein IIb/IIIa receptor is elevated.
- Bleeding time is prolonged in comparison to thrombocytopenia.

Bone marrow findings
- There is megakaryocyte hyperplasia with megakaryocytes having scant cytoplasm and hypolobated nucleus
- Bone marrow is not always required for diagnosis.

DISSEMINATED INTRAVASCULAR COAGULATION (DIC)

Definition: It is a serious fatal disorder which is characterized by widespread ischemic changes secondary to microvascular fibrin thrombi which are accompanied by consumption of platelets and coagulation factors leading to hemorrhagic diathesis.

Etiology: Causes of DIC include:

- Obstetric causes
  - Abruptio placenta
  - Retained dead fetus
  - Septic abortion
  - Amniotic fluid embolism
  - Toxemia
- Infections
  - Gram-negative sepsis
  - Meningococcemia
  - Rocky mountain spotted fever
  - Malaria
  - Histoplasmosis
- Massive tissue injury
  - Trauma
  - Burns
  - Extensive surgery
- Neoplasms
  - Pancreatic carcinoma
  - Acute promyelocytic leukemia
  - Prostate carcinoma.

Morphology

- Thrombi are found in brain, heart, lungs, kidneys, adrenals, spleen and liver in decreasing order of frequency
- Thrombi produce microinfarcts in various organs
- Erythrocytes are fragmented (schistocytes) due to passage through fibrin thrombi
- Platelet counts are reduced
- Depletion of clotting factors result in prolonged prothrombin time (PT), activated partial thromboplastin time (APTT), decreased plasma fibrinogen levels and increased plasma fibrin split products levels.

DISSEMINATED INTRAVASCULAR COAGULATION (DIC) (contd.)

Pathophysiology

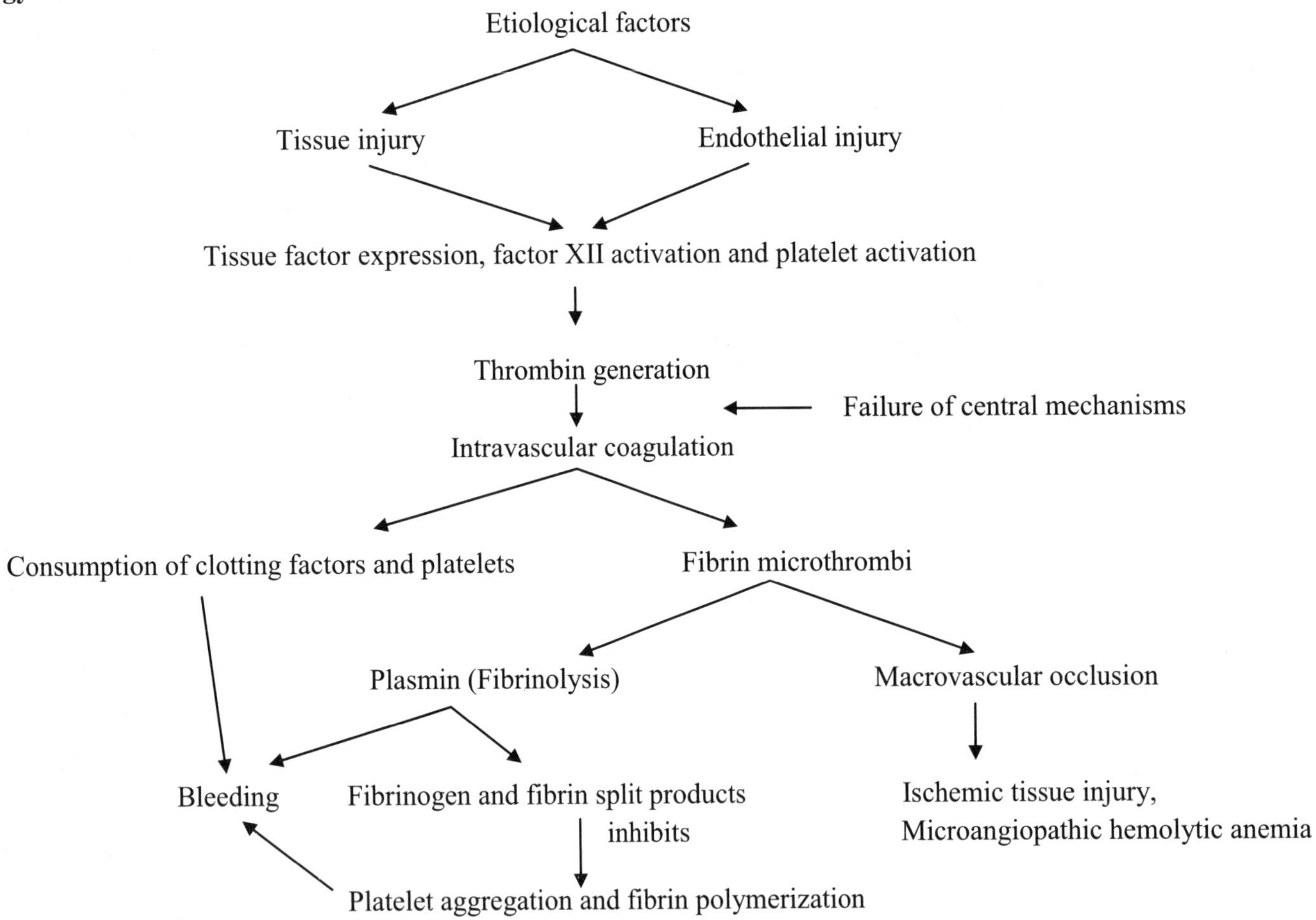

ATHEROSCLEROSIS

Definition: It is a disease of large and medium sized elastic muscular arteries that result in progressive accumulation within intima of inflammatory cells, smooth muscle cells, lipid and connective tissue.

Development

Fatty dot
↓
Fatty streak
↓
Intermediate lesion
↓
Atheroma
↓
Fibroatheroma
↓
Complicated lesion

Complications

- Rupture
- Ulceration
- Hemorrhage
- Aneurysm formation

Etiology

Major risk factors

Modifiable

- Hyperlipidemia
- Cigarette smoking
- Hypertension
- Diabetes mellitus

Non-modifiable

- Age—40–60 yrs
- Sex—M > F
- Family history of diabetes mellitus and hypertension
- Genetic abnormalities in lipid metabolism.

Minor risk factors

Non-modifiable

- Obesity
- Type A personality
- Physical inactivity
- Postmenopausal estrogen deficiency

Modifiable

- Alcohol intake
- PUFA intake
- Vascular infections

Gross pathology

Parts of atheroma

- Cap
- Shoulder
- Necrotic core

Microscopy

- Cap – smooth muscle cells + extracellular matrix
- Shoulder – smooth muscle cells + Inflammatory cells
- Core – Lipid, cell debris, fibrin, plasma proteins

Locations

- Abdominal aorta – Most common location **(Image J)**
- Coronary artery
- Popliteal artery
- Internal carotid artery

Pathogenesis

Endothelial injury
↓
Endothelial dysfunction
↓
Adhesion of monocytes to endothelium and migration to intima
↓
Transformation to foam cells
↓
Accumulation of lipoproteins and oxidation
↓
Adhesion of platelets to endothelium
↓
Migration of smooth muscle cells from media to intima under effect of mediators released from platelets and macrophages
↓
Proliferation of smooth muscle cells
↓
Laying of collagen
↓
More lipid accumulation

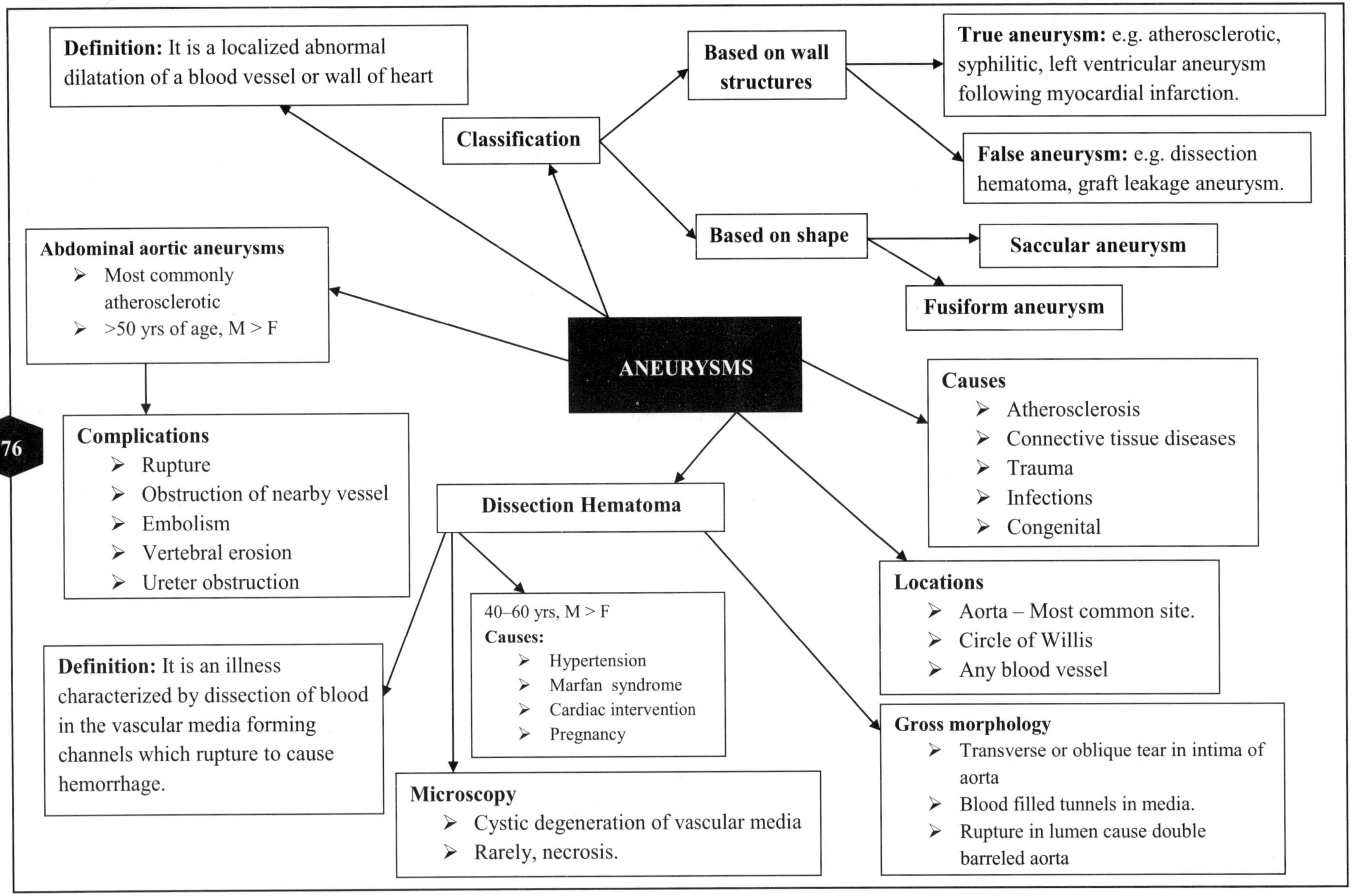
ANEURYSMS
Definition: It is a localized abnormal dilatation of a blood vessel or wall of heart
Classification
Based on wall structures
True aneurysm: e.g. atherosclerotic, syphilitic, left ventricular aneurysm following myocardial infarction.
False aneurysm: e.g. dissection hematoma, graft leakage aneurysm.
Based on shape
Saccular aneurysm
Fusiform aneurysm
Abdominal aortic aneurysms
➢ Most commonly atherosclerotic
➢ >50 yrs of age, M > F
Complications
➢ Rupture
➢ Obstruction of nearby vessel
➢ Embolism
➢ Vertebral erosion
➢ Ureter obstruction
Causes
➢ Atherosclerosis
➢ Connective tissue diseases
➢ Trauma
➢ Infections
➢ Congenital
Locations
➢ Aorta – Most common site.
➢ Circle of Willis
➢ Any blood vessel
Dissection Hematoma
Definition: It is an illness characterized by dissection of blood in the vascular media forming channels which rupture to cause hemorrhage.
40–60 yrs, M > F
Causes:
➢ Hypertension
➢ Marfan syndrome
➢ Cardiac intervention
➢ Pregnancy
Microscopy
➢ Cystic degeneration of vascular media
➢ Rarely, necrosis.
Gross morphology
➢ Transverse or oblique tear in intima of aorta
➢ Blood filled tunnels in media.
➢ Rupture in lumen cause double barreled aorta

VASCULITIDES

Definition: It is a group of vascular disorders characterized by inflammation of all layers of vessels wall

Classification

Based on etiology

Infectious vasculitis

- Bacterial
- Rickettsial
- Fungal
- Viral
- Spirochaetal

Immune vasculitis

Caused by immune complex deposits

- Henoch-Schönlein purpura
- Systemic lupus erythematosus
- Rheumatoid arthritis
- Cryoglobulinemia
- Serum sickness

Anti-neutrophilic cytoplasmic antibody (ANCA) mediated

- p – ANCA associated
- Microscopic polyangitis
- Churg-Strauss syndrome
- c – ANCA associated
- Wegener granulomatosis

Caused by antiendothelial antibodies

- Kawasaki disease
- Goodpasture syndrome

Based on vessels involved

Small vessel vasculitis

- Wegener granulomatosis
- Churg – Strauss syndrome
- Microscopic polyangitis

Medium vessel vasculitis

- Polyarteritis nodosa
- Kawasaki disease

Large vessel vasculitis

- Temporal arteritis
- Takayasu arteritis

Wegener granulomatosis

- Small vessel vasculitis characterised by triad of:
  - Necrotizing granulomas in upper respiratory tract
  - Granulomatous vasculitis of blood vessels.
  - Focal necrotizing or crescentic glomerulonephritis
- 40–50 yrs; M > F
- Associated with c - ANCA

Polyarteritis nodosa

- Medium vessel vasculitis affecting renal, visceral circulation and sparing pulmonary circulation
- 40–50 yrs, M > F
- Transmural necrotizing inflammation in all layers of vessel wall of all organs except lung.

Takayasu arteritis

- Pulseless disease
- < 40 yrs, F > M
- Similar to temporal arteritis in morphology
- Clinical features – diplopia, loss of vision, low blood pressure and weak pulse in upper extremities

Temporal arteritis

- It is a large vessel vasculitis affecting aorta, temporal, vertebral and ophthalmic artery characterized by necrotizing granulomas in blood vessels.
- > 60 yrs; M > F
- Grossly, nodular thickenings in blood vessels
- Microscopically, necrotizing granulomas in vascular media.
- Clinically, fever, weightloss, loss of vision, throbbing headache, diplopia and facial pain

HYPERTENSION (HTN)

Definition: It is a complex multisystem disease characterized by sustained elevation of systolic blood pressure >140 mm Hg or diastolic blood pressure >90 mm Hg

Classification

Based on clinical severity

Benign hypertension

- Systolic blood pressure >140 but <200 mm Hg
- Diastolic blood pressure >90 but <120 mm Hg

Malignant Hypertension

- Systolic blood pressure >200 mm Hg
- Diastolic blood pressure >120 mm Hg
- Renal failure
- Retinal exudates
- Poor prognosis

Based on etiology

Primary or essential hypertension (95%)

Secondary HTN (5%)

Cardiovascular causes

- Coarctation of aorta
- Increased cardiac output
- Rigid aorta

Neurologic causes

- Increased intracranial tension
- Sleep apnea
- Stress
- Psychogenic

Endocrine causes

- Cushing syndrome
- Conn syndrome
- Pheochromocytoma
- Acromegaly
- Hypothyroidism
- Hyperthyroidism
- Pregnancy

Renal causes

- Acute glomerulonephritis
- Chronic renal disease
- Polycystic kidney disease
- Renal artery stenosis
- Renal vasculitis
- Renin producing tumor
- Barrter syndrome
- Gitelman syndrome
- Liddle syndrome

Vascular pathology

Hyaline arteriosclerosis

- Seen in benign hypertension

Hyperplastic arteriosclerosis

- Seen in malignant hypertension

CONGENITAL HEART DISEASES

Definition: They are disorders affecting heart and great blood vessels which are present since birth.

Etiology

Genetic factors
- Increased incidence in trisomy 21, 18, 13, 15 and Turner syndrome

Environmental factors
- Viral infections – TORCH, HIV
- Drugs – Thalidomide, Warfarin, alcohol, Methotrexate, vitamin A
- Maternal diseases – Diabetes mellitus, phenylketonuria, etc.
- Radiation

Pathogenesis
- Mutations in transcription factor TBX5 gene associated with syndromic ASD and VSD
- Mutations in NKX2.5 causes nonsyndromic ASD
- Del. chromosome 22q11.2 associated with conotruncus abnormalities.

Classification (based on type of shunt)

L → R shunt
- ASD
- VSD
- Patent ductus arteriosus
- Patent truncus arteriosus
- Total anomalous pulmonary venous connection.

R → L shunt
- Tetrology of Fallot
- Tricuspid atresia

No shunt
- Transposition of great vessels
- Coarctation of aorta
- Pulmonary stenosis
- Aortic stenosis
- Ebstein anomaly
- Complete heart block.

Ventricular septal defect (VSD)
- Defect due to incomplete closure of ventricular septum
- 30% isolated; 70% cases associated with other abnormalities most commonly tetrology of Fallot
- 3 types (based on size, number and location)
  - Membranous VSD – 90% cases; defect in membranous septum
  - Muscular VSD – 5% cases defect in muscular part of septum; single to multiple (= Swiss cheese septum); spontaneous closure, thus, better prognosis.
  - Infundibular VSD – 5% cases defect located below pulmonary valve.

Atrial septal defect (ASD)
- Most common congenital heart disease; asymptomatic till adulthood.
- 3 types (based on location of defect in atrial septum)
  - Secundum ASD – Defect in middle part of septum; 95%
  - Primum ASD – Defect in atrial septum above atrioventricular valve; 5%
  - Sinus venosus ASD – Defect in atrial septum just below superior vena cava opening.

HEART FAILURE

Definition: It is the inability to maintain normal cardiac output that is adequate for tissue metabolic needs despite normal venous return.

Classification

Based on duration of development

Acute heart failure

- Occurs within hours to few days
- Causes – Acute coronary artery occlusion, pulmonary embolism, malignant hypertension
- Complications – Pulmonary edema, brain and renal ischemia; sudden death

Chronic heart failure

- Occurs in weeks to months
- Causes – Severe anemia, chronic valvular disease, chronic lung disease, hypertension
- Complications – Chronic venous congestion lung, liver; long-standing edema.

Based on side of heart involved

Right ventricular failure (Corpulmonale)

- Causes – Chronic lung disease, mitral stenosis, secondary to left ventricular failure
- Morphological changes– chronic venous congestion liver, spleen; ascites; congestive nephropathy; pleural effusion; pericardial effusion; anasarca

Left ventricular failure

- Causes – Ischemic heart disease, systemic hypertension, Mitral regurgitation, aortic stenosis.
- Morphological changes – Chronic venous congestion lung, ischemic nephropathy, hypoxic encephalopathy.

Based on cardiac output

Low output cardiac failure

- Inability to maintain normal cardiac output
- Cardiac output < 4 L/minute
- Causes – Hypertension, ischemic heart disease, valvular heart disease, myocarditis.

High output cardiac failure

- Inability to maintain abnormally high cardiac output
- Cardiac output >6 L/minute
- Causes – Chronic anemia, hyperthyroidism, atrioventricular shunting

ISCHEMIC HEART DISEASE (IHD)

Definition: It is a group of closely related syndromes resulting from myocardial ischemia.

Etiology
- Systemic hypertension
- Cigarette smoking
- Diabetes mellitus
- Obesity
- Old age
- Sex: M > F
- Family history
- Oral contraceptive pill usage: Females >35 yrs on these pills have very high-risk
- Type A personality
- Sedentary lifestyle

Pathogenesis
- Diminished coronary blood flow as compared to myocardial demand due to atheroma with secondary changes, intraluminal thrombosis, platelet aggregation and vasospasm.

Classification

Angina pectoris: It is a type of IHD characterized by substernal chest discomfort caused by transient myocardial ischemia that falls short of causing infarction.

Types
- **Stable or typical angina:** It occurs due to decreased coronary blood flow secondary to atherosclerosis.
- **Unstable or atypical angina:** Occurs due to disruption of atheroma with superimposed thrombus
- **Prinzmetal or variant angina** Occurs due to coronary vasospasm

Myocardial infarction

Sudden cardiac death

Ischemic heart disease with congestive cardiac failure

MYOCARDIAL INFARCTION (MI)

Definition: It is defined as the death of cardiac muscle secondary to ischemia.

Sites of infarction based on blood vessels involved

Right coronary artery (30 – 40% cases)
- Posterior wall of left ventricle
- Posterior part of interventricular septum

Left anterior descending branch of left coronary artery (40–50% cases)
- Anterior wall of left ventricle
- Anterior part of interventricular septum
- Apex of heart

Left circumflex coronary artery (15–20% cases)
- Lateral wall of left ventricle except apex of heart

Types

Transmural infarct
- Involves entire thickness of muscle wall.
- Unifocal; solid
- Occurs in distribution of specific coronary artery
- Complications – Shock, epicarditis, aneurysm

Subendocardial infarct
- Involves inner one-third or half of ventricular wall.
- Multifocal; Patchy
- No epicarditis
- No aneurysm formation
- Coronary thrombosis is

Prognosis
- Depends on –
  - Infarct size – larger infarct; poor prognosis.
  - Infarct site – anterior wall MI has worser prognosis
  - Infarct type – transmural infarcts have worser prognosis as compared to subendocardial infarcts.

Complications
- Contractile dysfunction
- Sinus bradycardia
- Ventricular asystole
- Ventricular tachycardia
- Ventricular fibrillation
- Complete heart block.
- Rupture of ventricular free wall
- Rupture of ventricular septum
- Papillary muscle rupture
- Pericarditis
- Right ventricular infarction
- Ventricular aneurysm
- Papillary muscle dysfunction
- Late heart failure.

Serological enzymes markers
- Troponin T and I levels –
  - Most sensitive marker; absent normally
  - Increases 2 – 4 hrs after infarct, peak at 48 hrs and elevated till 7–10 days.
- Creatine kinase –
  - 3 isoenzymes – CK-MM, MB and BB
  - CK-MB is most sensitive
  - Increases 2–4 hrs after infarct, peak at 24 hours and normal in 72 hours
- C – reactive protein (CRP) –
  - > 3 mg/l associated with high-risk of cardiovascular disease.

Microscopic morphological changes
- First 24 hours – coagulative necrosis begins 4 – 12 hours after attack, myocyte hypereosinophilia, nuclear pyknosis, neutrophilic infiltrate begins.
- 2 – 3 days – accumulation of neutrophils at periphery of necrotic muscle fibres, muscle fibres show reduced striation.
- 5 – 7 days – neutrophils abate, macrophage and lymphocytes accumulate, fibroblasts lay collagen from 5th day.
- 1 – 3 weeks – collagen deposition, inflammation recedes, sprouted capillaries are well formed.
- > 4 weeks – dense fibrous tissue with less cellular scar.

Gross morphological changes (Image K)
- First 24 hours – dark brown mottling seen.
- 2–3 days – dark mottling with yellow tan centre
- 1–3 weeks – red grey depressed infarct with gelatinous appearance.
- More than 4 weeks – grey white scar formation from periphery to center.
- 5–8 weeks – complete grey white scarring

VEGETATIONS IN HEART

Definition: They are small to large thickenings in the endocardium composed of fibrin, erythrocytes and inflammatory cells.

Types

Infected vegetations

Infective endocarditis: It is the infection of mural endocardium leading to formation of bulky, friable vegetations containing microbes associated with destruction of underlying cardiac tissue.

Classification (based on severity of disease)
- Acute endocarditis—highly virulent organism (*Staphylococcus aureus, Streptococcus pyogenes*) infection of previously normal valve with death within days to weeks.
- Subacute endocarditis—low virulence (*Streptococcus viridans* and *Staphylococcus epidermidis*) organism infection of previously deformed cardiac valves with very less chance of death.

Etiology
- **High-risk individuals**
  - Myxomatous mitral valve
  - Calcific valve stenosis
  - Bicuspid aortic valve
  - Prosthetic valve
  - Neutropenia
  - Immunodeficiency
  - Malignancy
  - Diabetes mellitus
  - Alcohol abuse
  - Intravenous drug abuse
- **Pathogenic organisms**
  - *Staphylococcus aureus*
  - *Streptococcus pyogenes*
  - *Staphylococcus epidermidis*
  - HACEK group of bacteria
  - Fungi
  - Chlamydia
  - Rickettsiae.

Morphology
- Single to multiple, friable, bulky vegetations on atrioventricular valves and endocardium of chambers. **(Image L)**
- Ring abscess—vegetations erode the myocardium and form circular abscess.
- Large, less destructive vegetations in fungal endocarditis.
- Vegetations are composed of inflammatory cells, fibrin, RBCs and microbes.

VEGETATIONS IN HEART (contd.)

Types (contd.)

Non-infected vegetations

- **Rheumatic fever:** It is a multisystem disease which follows a streptococcal pharyngitis and is characterized by inflammation of heart, joints and central nervous system

Etiopathogenesis

- Type III hypersensitivity; antibodies formed against M protein of streptococcus cross react with glycoproteins in heart, joints and central nervous system

Morphology

- Pancarditis—inflammation of all 3 layers of heart.
- Endocardium—vegetation 1–2 mm along the line of closure of valves; Maccallum fibrous plaque in left atrium.
- Myocardium—Aschoff's nodule compound of Anitschkow cells, lymphocytes, multinucleated giant cells and fibroblasts.
- Pericardium—serofibrinous pericarditis (= bread and butter pericarditis)
- Chronic rheumatic heart disease—fibrosis replaces inflammation with valvular leaflet thickening and commissural fusion causing fish-mouth or button hole mitral valve stenosis.

Complications

- Congestive heart failure
- Mural thrombus
- Infective endocarditis
- Adhesive pericarditis.

Clinical features (Modified Jones criteria for diagnosis)

- 2 major or 1 major + 2 minor for diagnosis
- Major manifestations—carditis, subcutaneous nodules, erythema marginatum, Sydenham chorea, migratory polyarthritis of large joints
- Major manifestations—fever, arthralgia, increased erythrocyte sedimentation rate, increased C—reactive protein, leucocytosis, previous history of rheumatic fever.

Non-bacterial thrombotic endocarditis

- Also known as Marantic endocarditis
- Causes—mucinous adenocarcinoma of pancreas, acute myeloid leukemia—M4, sepses, wasting diseases, burns, hyperestrogenic states, cardiovascular intervention.
- Morphology—sterile (1–5 mm) vegetations along the line of closure of valves or valve cusps.

Libman-Sack endocarditis

- Also known as systemic lupus erythematosus endocarditis
- 1–4 mm multiple vegetations on undersurface of valves, cords, valvular endocardium and chambers
- Microscopically, vegetations contain hematoxylin or LE bodies.

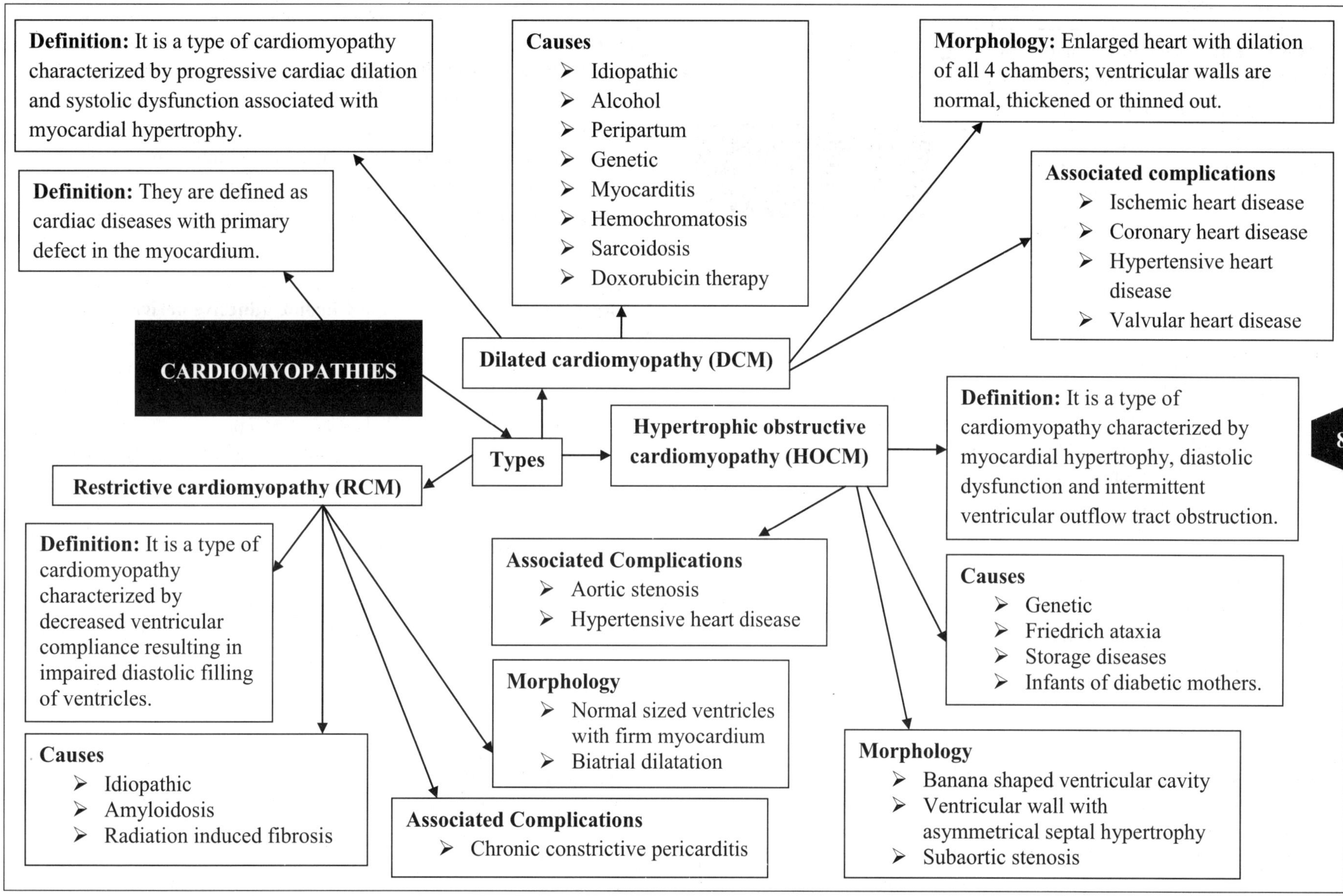
CARDIOMYOPATHIES
Definition: They are defined as cardiac diseases with primary defect in the myocardium.
Types
Dilated cardiomyopathy (DCM)
Definition: It is a type of cardiomyopathy characterized by progressive cardiac dilation and systolic dysfunction associated with myocardial hypertrophy.
Causes
➢ Idiopathic
➢ Alcohol
➢ Peripartum
➢ Genetic
➢ Myocarditis
➢ Hemochromatosis
➢ Sarcoidosis
➢ Doxorubicin therapy
Morphology: Enlarged heart with dilation of all 4 chambers; ventricular walls are normal, thickened or thinned out.
Associated complications
➢ Ischemic heart disease
➢ Coronary heart disease
➢ Hypertensive heart disease
➢ Valvular heart disease
Hypertrophic obstructive cardiomyopathy (HOCM)
Definition: It is a type of cardiomyopathy characterized by myocardial hypertrophy, diastolic dysfunction and intermittent ventricular outflow tract obstruction.
Causes
➢ Genetic
➢ Friedrich ataxia
➢ Storage diseases
➢ Infants of diabetic mothers.
Associated Complications
➢ Aortic stenosis
➢ Hypertensive heart disease
Morphology
➢ Banana shaped ventricular cavity
➢ Ventricular wall with asymmetrical septal hypertrophy
➢ Subaortic stenosis
Restrictive cardiomyopathy (RCM)
Definition: It is a type of cardiomyopathy characterized by decreased ventricular compliance resulting in impaired diastolic filling of ventricles.
Causes
➢ Idiopathic
➢ Amyloidosis
➢ Radiation induced fibrosis
Associated Complications
➢ Chronic constrictive pericarditis
Morphology
➢ Normal sized ventricles with firm myocardium
➢ Biatrial dilatation

PERICARDITIS

Definition: It is the inflammation of pericardium due to external causes with no primary defect in the pericardium.

Causes
- Infectious agents—bacteria, viruses, fungus, tuberculosis (TB), parasites like Trypanosoma.
- Immune mediated—rheumatic fever, systemic lupus erythematosus (SLE), postmyocardial infarction (Dressler syndrome), systemic sclerosis.
- Miscellaneous—MI, uremia, trauma, radiation, cardiac intervention.

Classification

Acute pericarditis

Acute hemorrhagic pericarditis
- Causes—Tumors, TB, bleeding diathesis, postcardiac surgery.
- Blood mixed serous or fibrinous fluid accumulated in pericardial sac.

Acute purulent pericarditis
- Causes—Bacterial infection
- 400–500 ml pus in pericardial sac; red granular surface of pericardium.

Acute caseous pericarditis
- Cause—TB
- Grey white, cheese like material accumulated in pericardial sac.

Acute serous pericarditis
- Causes—Noninfectious inflammation, tumors, uremia.
- 50–200 ml serous fluid accumulates in pericardial sac.
- Microscopically, inflammatory infiltrate comprising neutrophils, lymphocytes and macrophages seen.

Acute fibrinous pericarditis
- Causes—Post-MI, uremia, chest radiation, rheumatic fever, SLE
- Thick, creamy fluid in pericardial sac; dry pericardium with fine granular roughening.

Chronic pericarditis

Chronic adhesive pericarditis
- Causes—Post-TB, Post-cardiac intervention, post-radiation, postbacterial infection.
- Dense adhesions between 2 layers of pericardium.

Chronic constrictive pericarditis
- Resembles RCM
- No specific cause known
- Limited diastolic expansion of ventricles due to fibrocalcific scar in pericardium.

SALIVARY GLAND TUMORS

Benign tumors

- Oncocytoma
- Ductal papilloma
- Basal cell adenoma
- Canalicular adenoma

Pleomorphic adenoma (Benign mixed tumor) (Fig. 33)

- It is the most common tumor of salivary gland is a benign neoplasm characterized by biphasic appearance which is an admixture of epithelial and stromal elements.
- Comprise 50 – 60% of parotid tumor
- Rare in submandibular and minor salivary glands.
- Gross morphology—Well-demarcated rounded masses upto 6 cm in size.
- Microscopy—Encapsulated masses; epithelial elements composed of ductal and myoepithelial cells arranged in acini, ducts, tubules and cords; mesenchymal component composed of myxoid tissue with islands of cartilage and bone.

Warthin tumor (Papillary cystadenoma lymphomatosum) (Fig. 34)

- It is a benign neoplasm of parotid composed of cystic glandular spaces embedded in dense lymphoid tissue.
- Second most common benign salivary neoplasm
- M > F; 5th to 7th decade
- 10% multifocal; 10% bilateral
- Gross morphology – Round to oval, pale grey encapsulated masses 3 – 4 cm in size and has cleft like spaces on cut surface.
- Microscopy – spaces are lined by double layered neoplastic epithelial cells with dense lymphoid stroma. The surface epithelium show columnar cells with abundant finely granular, eosinophilic cytoplasm (oncocytes). The inner layer is composed of polygonal or cuboidal cells.

Malignant tumors

- Malignant mixed tumors
- Acinic cell tumor
- Adenocarcinoma
- Adenoid cystic carcinoma
- Squamous cell carcinoma

Mucoepidermoid carcinoma

- It is a malignant salivary gland tumor composed of a mixture of neoplastic squamous cells, mucus secreting cells and epithelial cells of intermediate type.
- Most common malignant salivary gland tumor
- 60–70% in parotid;
- Gross morphology—3–7 cm, well-circumscribed but unencapsulated grey white tumors with mucin filled cysts.
- Microscopy—Cords, sheets and cysts of squamous, mucous and intermediate cells.

PEPTIC ULCER DISEASE

Definition: They are chronic, most often solitary breaks in the mucosa of stomach or small intestine or lower gastrointestinal tract due to aggressive action of acid peptic juices.

Microscopy (Fig. 35): 4 zones seen in active ulcers—(from surface below)
- Superficial thin layer of fibrinoid necrosis.
- Layer with inflammatory cells predominantly neutrophils
- Granulation tissue layer with mononuclear leukocytes.
- Solid fibrous or collagenous scar.

Gross morphology
- Age—Middle aged to older adults
- Sex—Duodenal ulcer M:F::3:1
  Gastric ulcer M: F::1.5 – 2:1
- Duodenum and stomach – most common site in ratio of 4:1
- Duodenal ulcer—More commonly on anterior wall.
- Gastric ulcer—Along lesser curvature between body and pylorus
- Grossly, ulcer is round to oval with straight walls and punched out margins. Base of ulcer is smooth and clear
- Mucosa surrounding the ulcer appears to be radiating like spokes of a wheel.

Complications
- Bleeding—most common complication
- Perforation
- Obstruction due to fibrosis.

Pathogenesis
- Imbalance between gastroduodenal mucosal defense mechanism and damaging forces.
- Defensive forces are:
  - Surface mucous secretion
  - Bicarbonate secretion in mucous
  - Prostaglandins
  - Mucosal blood flow
  - Epithelial regenerative capacity
- Damaging forces are:
  - Gastric acidity
  - Peptic enzymes
- Role of *Helicobacter pylori* infection:
  - It induces inflammation and immune response
  - Urease from *Helicobacter pylori* forms toxic components like NH_4Cl which cause epithelial injury.
  - It enhances gastric acid secretion and inhibits HCO_3 secretion.

Locations: (in decreasing order of frequency)
- First part of duodenum
- Antrum of stomach
- Gastroesophageal junction
- Margins of gastrojejunostomy
- Ectopic gastric mucosa in ileal Meckel diverticulum

Etiology
- Diet—Spicy food and caffeine are ulcerogenic
- Drugs—Aspirin and other non-steroidal anti-inflammatory drugs inhibit prostaglandins and cause ulcers.
- Cigarette smoking—It impairs mucosal blood flow and healing.
- Alcohol—Alcoholic cirrhosis is associated with increased incidence of peptic ulcers.
- Family history— First degree relatives have 3 times higher risk.
- *Helicobacter pylori* infection—It is seen in all cases with duodenal ulcer and 70% cases of gastric ulcers.
- Blood group antigens—Persons with 'O' blood group have 30% higher risk of duodenal ulcers than those with group A, B, AB.
- Chronic obstructive pulmonary disease
- Chronic renal failure and hyperparathyioidism—Hypercalcemia stimulates gastrin and acid production
- Gastric hyperacidity and duodenogastric reflux—It is highly ulcerogenic.

GASTRIC CARCINOMA

Definition: It is the most common malignant tumor of stomach
- Age—5th – 7th decade
- M:F::2:1

Pathogenesis: Allelic loss of several genes e.g. TGFβ, p53, BAX etc. leads to tumorigenesis.

Etiological factors
- Environmental factors:
  - Alcohol intake
  - Nitrites derived from nitrates in water
  - Smoked food
  - Starchy food, pickles
  - Lack of fruits
  - Smoking
  - Low socioeconomic status
  - *H. pylori* infection
- Host factors:
  - Partial gastrectomy
  - Chronic gastritis
  - Gastric adenomas
  - Barret esophagus
- Genetic factors:
  - Blood group A individuals
  - Family history
  - Hereditary non-polyposis colon carcinoma syndrome

Classification

Lauren classification— (2 subtypes)
- Intestinal type – Bulky tumors with malignant cells in diffuse sheet and glandular pattern
  - Age—55yrs; M:F::2:1
- Diffuse type—Malignant cell in diffuse sheets
  - Age—48 yrs; M:F::1:1

WHO classification
- Epithelial tumors
  - Adenoma
  - Adenocarcinoma
    - Mucinous adenocarcinoma
    - Tubular adenocarcinoma
    - Papillary adenocarcinoma
    - Signet ring cell adenocarcinoma
    - Adenosquamous carcinoma.
  - Small cell carcinoma
  - Carcinoid
- Non-epithelial tumors
  - Leiomyoma
  - Schwannoma
  - Granular cell tumor
  - Leiomyosarcoma
  - Kaposi sarcoma
  - Lymphoma

Gross morphology
- Location—Pylorus and antrum (60–65% cases); cardia (25–30% cases); rest in body and fundus.
- Lesser curvature involved in 40% cases while greater curvature in 15% cases.
- Most common location—lesser curvature of antropyloric region
- Macroscopic growth patterns
  - Exophytic
  - Flat or depressed
  - Excavated
- Linitus plastic—Leather bottle appearance due to complete infiltration of stomach wall by tumor. **(Image M)**

Microscopy (Fig. 36)
- 2 histological subtypes
  - Intestinal type—neoplastic glands with expanding growth pattern and cells having mucin vacuoles
  - Diffuse type—neoplastic cells are in singles or small clusters and have large mucin vacuole in cytoplasm pushing the nucleus to periphery (signet ring appearance)

INFLAMMATORY BOWEL DISEASE (IBD)

Definition: It is a set of chronic inflammatory conditions resulting from excessive activation of intestinal mucosal immune system in response to normal intraluminal flora.

Etiopathogenesis

- Two major pathogenic changes are:
  - Strong immune response against normal intestinal flora in genetically susceptible individual
  - Defect in epithelial barrier function.
- Genetic susceptibility:
  - First degree relatives have two times higher risk than general population.
  - Monozygotic twins have 30–40% risk of developing IBD.
  - HLADR1 is associated with 27% cases of Crohn disease; HLADR2 is seen in 20% cases of ulcerative colitis.
- Role of intestinal flora:
  - Defects in epithelial barrier allow entry of microbes and activation of mucosal immune system.
- Abnormal T-cell response:
  - Exaggerated T-cell activation or abnormal T-cell regulation cause immune injury to gut wall.

Classification

Ulcerative colitis

Gross morphology (Image N)

- Pancolitis—It begins in rectum and progresses retrograde to involve entire colon.
- Backwash ileitis—In severe pancolitis, distal ileum develops diffuse mucosal inflammation.
- Appendiceal involvement may be seen.
- Pseudopolyps—The regenerating mucosa in between the diseased mucosa bulges outwards to form pseudopolyps
- Toxic megacolon—In severe cases, muscularis propria and neural axis is affected causing dilated colon.

Definition: It is an ulceroinflammatory disease limited to the colon affecting only mucous and submucosa and is characterized by chronic diarrhea and rectal bleeding with a pattern of exacerbations and remissions with a possibility of serious complications.

Microscopy

- Continuous mucosal involvement with no skip lesions.
- Crypt abscesses and mononuclear inflammatory infiltrate in lamina propria
- No granulomas noted.
- No serositis or fistulae formation noted.

INFLAMMATORY BOWEL DISEASE (IBD) (contd.)

Classification (contd.)

Crohn disease

Definition: It is a transmural chronic inflammatory disease that may affect any part of digestive tract principally distal small intestine and right colon with presence of non-caseating granulomas and followed by fissuring and fistula formation.

Gross morphology (Image O)

- Small intestine is involved in 40–45% cases; small intestine and colon in 25–30% cases and colon alone in 25% cases.
- It may rarely involve any part of gut from esophagus to anal canal
- The involved bowel segment is edematous thick and rubbery
- Surrounding mesenteric fat wraps around involved bowel (creeping fat)
- Skip lesions – Sharp demarcation between diseased and adjacent uninvolved bowel segment
- Cobble stone appearance of mucosa due to swelling, fibrosis and ulceration
- Fissuring and fistula formation is commonly seen.

Microscopic features

- Mucosal neutrophilic inflammation with formation of crypt abscesses
- Mucosal damage characterized by villous blunting, crypt irregularity and branching
- Mucosal ulceration
- Transmural chronic inflammation upto serosa
- Non-caseating granulomas in all layers of involved as well as uninvolved regions of bowel wall in 30 – 50% cases
- Transmural fibrosis leading to stricture formation
- Mucosal and submucosal lymphangiectasia
- Hypertrophy of mural nerve fibres.

MALABSORPTION SYNDROMES

Definition: It is a group of disorders characterized by inadequate absorption of important nutrients by the gastrointestinal tract.

Classification: (Based on defective digestion and intestinal tract abnormalities)

- Defect in luminal digestion
  - Pancreatic insufficiency
  - Zollinger-Ellison syndrome
  - Ileal dysfunction
  - Bile flow obstruction
  - Hepatic dysfunction
- Mucosal abnormality
  - Abetalipoproteinemia
  - Bacterial overgrowth syndrome
  - Lactose intolerance
- Lymphatic obstruction
  - Tuberculosis
  - Malignant tumors
- Reduced surface area of intestinal absorptive zone.
  - Celiac disease
  - Crohn disease
- Infections
  - Tropical sprue
  - Whipple disease
  - Parasitic enteritis
  - Bacterial enteritis
  - Viral enteritis.

Complications

- Anemia—due to vitamin B_{12} or iron deficiency
- Bleeding—due to led vitamin K absorption
- Tetany—due to calcium deficiency
- Amenorrhea, infertility
- Purpura, petechiae—due to vitamin K deficiency
- Dermatitis
- Edema
- Peripheral neuropathy
- Diarrhea, abdominal pain.

Celiac disease (Gluten sensitive enteropathy)

Definition: It is a chronic disease syndrome characterized by generalized malabsorption, small intestinal mucosal lesions and a prompt clinical and histopathological response to withdrawal of gluten containing food from diet.

Pathogenesis

- T-cell mediated immune response to alcohol soluble gliadin protein in wheat, barley, rye and oats.
- HLA DQ2 and DQ8 are closely associated with the disease.

Morphology

- Endoscopically, mucosa is flattened.
- Microscopically, diffuse enteritis with marked atrophy or total loss of villi.
- There is loss of microvilli
- Lamina contains increased lymphocytes.
- Crypts are elongated and hypertrophic.

MALABSORPTION SYNDROMES (contd.)

Whipple disease

Definition: It is a rare systemic disease principally affecting intestine, central nervous system and joints caused by bacterium *Trophyrema whippelii.*

Morphology

- Hallmark of disease is thickening of small intestinal villi due to presence of bacilli laden macrophages in the lamina propria.

Tropical sprue (Post-infectious sprue)

Definition: It is a celiac like disease occurring in tropical region most probably secondary to enterotoxic organism infections e.g. *Escherichia coli* and *Hemophilus.*

Morphology

- It involves any portion of intestine
- Microscopically, diffuse enteritis with villous atrophy and crypt hyperplasia noted.

COLORECTAL POLYPS

Definition: It is a tumorous mass that protrudes into the lumen of the gut.

Classification

Based on attachment to bowel wall
- Sessile
- Pedunculated.

Based on malignant potential
- Non-neoplastic polyp
- Neoplastic polyp

Based on histopathological appearance
- Hyperplastic polyp
- Serrated polyp
- Adenomatous polyp

Non-neoplastic polyps

Definition: They are polyps of gut which have no malignant potential.

Types

Hamartomatous polyps: They are polypoidal hamartomas of mucosal epithelium and lamina propria.

Subtypes

Cronkhite Canada syndrome
- Non-hereditary disorder characterized by:
  - Gastrointestinal hamartomatous polyps
  - Nail atrophy
  - Skin pigmentation
  - Alopecia.

Juvenile polyp (Fig. 37)
- Hamartomatous polyp in children less than 10 years
- Majority occur in rectum; rest in colon
- 1–3 cm, pedunculated retention polyp with cystically dilated glands and stroma.

Cowden syndrome
- Autosomal dominant
- Characterized by:
  - Intestinal hamartomatous polyps
  - Facial trichilemmoma
  - Acral keratosis
  - Oral papillomas.

Peutz-Jegher polyp
- Hamartomatous polyp with mucosal epithelium, lamina propria and muscularis mucosa
- Multiple; large, pedunculated polyps
- Location—Most commonly small intestine followed by colon and stomach
- Patients with these polyps have high-risk of malignancy of pancreas, breast, lung, ovary and uterus.

Inflammatory polyp
- They are not true neoplasms but rather elevated nodules of inflamed and regenerating epithelium.

Lymphoid polyp
- They are submucosal accumulations of lymphoid tissue invariably in rectum which are seen as single sessile nodule measuring upto 5 cm in diameter.

Hyperplastic polyp
- They are small sessile mucosal excrescences that display exaggerated crypt architecture.
- Single to multiple; majority in rectum and sigmoid colon.

COLORECTAL POLYPS (contd.)

Neoplastic polyps (Adenomatous polyps)

Definition: They are polyps arising from mucosal epithelium and have malignant potential.

Hereditary nonpolyposis colorectal cancer syndrome
- Autosomal dominant inheritance
- Increased risk of colorectal cancer and endometrial carcinoma.

Familial adenomatous polyposis (FAP) syndrome
- Caused by mutation in APC gene on chromosome 5q21
- Classification:
    - Classic FAP: 500–2500 polyps, majority being tubular adenoma.
    - Attenuated FAP—fewer polyp, majority in proximal colon
    - Gardner syndrome—Classic FAP, osteomas, fibromas, epidermal cysts
    - Turcot syndrome—Classic FAP, CNS tumors e.g. Medulloblastoma and glioblastoma multiforme.

Subtypes (Based on epithelial architecture)

Tubulovillous adenoma
- Adenomas with >25% and <75% villous architecture.

Tubular adenoma
- Most common adenoma.
- They are smooth surfaced lesions < 2 cm in diameter and have a stalk; smaller ones are sessile.
- Location—Majority in colon; rest in stomach and small intestine.
- They comprise two-thirds of adenomas.
- Microscopically, closely packed epithelial tubules are embedded in fibrovascular stroma.

Villous adenoma
- Sessile, cauliflower like masses 1–3 cm above the surface
- Location—rectum and rectosigmoid colon
- Microscopically, finger like projections lined by tall columnar epithelium seen.
- Higher malignant potential than tubular adenoma.

COLORECTAL CARCINOMA

Definition: They are malignant tumor of the large intestine, adenocarcinoma in majority of cases.

- Age—60–80 years.
- Sex—Males : Females : : 1.5 : 1

Microscopic features

- Tumors of both right and left colon have similar features
- They are well to poorly differentiated adenocarcinomas with strong desmoplastic response.

Gross morphology (Image P)

- Most common location of cancer is rectosigmoid followed by cecum.
- Cancers in proximal colon are exophytic, polypoid masses.
- Cancers in distal colon are annular, encircling lesions producing napkin ring constrictions.

Etiology: Major risk factors include

- Excess dietary animal fat
- Deficient dietary intake of unabsorbable fibres
- High content of refined carbohydrates
- Low intake of antioxidants, e.g. vitamin E, A, C
- Low intake of cruciferous vegetables, e.g. cauliflower, cabbage
- Ulcerative colitis and Crohn disease.

Pathogenesis: There are two pathogenetically distinct pathways of colorectal carcinogenesis.

- Microsatellite instability pathway
  - Genetic lesions in DNA mismatch repair genes cause accumulation of mutations in microsatellites that are involved in genes causing cell growth regulation such as TGF-β and BAX genes.

- APC/β-catenin pathway
  - It is characterized by chromosomal instability leading to step wise accumulation of mutations in oncogenes and antioncogenes.
  - The genetic correlates of this pathway are as follows:

Loss of APC gene on chromosome 5q

↓

Mutation of K – RAS gene

↓

Loss of SMAD on chromosome 18q

↓

Loss of p53 on chromosome 17p

↓

Activation of telomerase.

CIRRHOSIS

Definition: It is the end stage of chronic liver disease defined as the destruction of normal hepatic architecture by fibrous septae that encompasses regenerative nodules of hepatocytes. **(Fig. 38)**

Etiology

- Alcoholic liver disease (Most common cause)
- Chronic viral hepatitis.
- Primary biliary cirrhosis
- Autoimmune hepatitis
- Extrahepatic biliary obstruction
- Primary sclerosing cholangitis
- Hemochromatosis
- Wilson disease
- Cystic fibrosis
- α_1-antitrypsin deficiency
- Glycogen storage disorders
- Idiopathic

Classification
(Based on the size of nodules)

Micronodular cirrhosis

- In this type, the nodules are < 3 mm in diameter
- It is seen in alcoholic cirrhosis.

Macronodular cirrhosis (Image Q)

- In this type, the nodules are > 3 mm in diameter
- It is classically seen in chronic hepatitis.

Pathogenesis: The pathogenetic process includes:

- Progressive fibrosis
- Reorganization of vascular microarchitecture of liver
- Excess collagen during fibrosis is produced by perisinusoidal stellate cells that undergo myofibroblast transformation and produce extracellular collagen matrix.
- Stellate cell activation and transformation occurs under the influence of tumor necrosis factor, interleukin-1 and TGF-β released from endothelial cells, Kupffer cells and inflammatory cells.

CIRRHOSIS (contd.)

Complications
- Hepatic failure
- Portal hypertension
- Hepatopulmonary syndrome
- Hepatorenal syndrome
- Hepatocellular carcinoma.

Hepatic failure

Definition: It is a clinical syndrome that occurs when a mass of liver cells or their function is inadequate to sustain metabolic, detoxifying and synthetic activity of the liver.

Consequences
- Cholestasis and jaundice
- Hyperalbuminemia
- Hypoglycemia
- Gynecomastia
- Hypogonadism
- Weightloss
- Hyperammonemia.

Life-threatning complications
- Coagulopathy – due to reduced synthesis of coagulation factors.
- Hepatic encephalopathy
- Multiorgan failure.

Portal hypertension

Definition: It is defined as sustained increase in portal venous pressure resulting from obstruction in portal circuit
- Portal vein pressure >30 mm H_2O is considered portal hypertension.

Clinical consequences
- Ascites
- Portosystemic shunts
- Congestive splenomegaly
- Hepatic encephalopathy.

Etiology: Based on the site of obstruction of portal blood flow
- Prehepatic:
  - Portal vein thrombosis
- Intrahepatic:
  - Cirrhosis
  - Sarcoidosis
  - Schistosomiasis
  - Primary biliary cirrhosis
  - Congenital hepatic fibrosis
  - Toxins e.g. Arsenic.

ALCOHOLIC LIVER DISEASE

Definition: It is a chronic disorder with overlapping morphological and clinical entities which include:
- Hepatic steatosis
- Alcoholic hepatitis and
- Cirrhosis.

Pathogenesis
- Short-term ingestion of 70–90 grams of alcohol over several days produce fatty liver
- Daily intake of >150g of alcohol for 10–20 years is associated with severe hepatic injury
- Alcohol induces defects in fatty acid catabolism and bifurcates it to cause lipid biosynthesis
- Alcohol induces impaired hepatic metabolism of methionine sensitizing the liver to oxidative injury
- Alcohol induces cytochrome P450 enzyme leading to production of free radicals causing toxic injury to hepatocytes.

Morphology

Alcoholic cirrhosis
- Grossly, liver is brown and shrunken
- Microscopically, formation of nodules and fibrosis occurs. **(Fig. 38)**

Hepatic steatosis
- Moderate intake of alcohol causes microvescular steatosis
- Chronic intake causes macrovesicular steatosis.

Alcoholic hepatitis
- Hepatocyte swelling and necrosis
- Mallory bodies—Accumulation of cytokeratin as eosinophilic inclusions in degenerating hepatocytes
- Periportal and perivenular fibrosis
- Inflammation surrounding degenerated hepatocytes.

VIRAL HEPATITIS

Definition: It is a viral infection of hepatocytes that produce necrosis and inflammation of the liver.

Etiology

- Hepatitis A virus
- Hepatitis B virus
- Hepatitis C virus
- Hepatitis E virus
- Yellow fever virus
- Epstein-Barr virus
- Lassa virus
- Ebola virus
- Marburg virus
- Herpes simplex virus
- Cytomegalovirus

Clinicopathological syndrome

- Acute asymptomatic infection with recovery
- Acute symptomatic infection
  - Anicteric phase
  - Icteric phase
- Chronic hepatitis
  - Without or with progressions to cirrhosis
  - Fuminant hepatitis.

Morphology

Chronic hepatitis

- Portal lymphohistiocytic inflammation with destruction of bile ducts
- Mild to moderate marcovesicular steatosis
- Interface hepatitis
- Periportal septal fibrosis
- Bridging fibrosis.

Fulminant hepatitis

- Grossly, liver is a limp, red and covered by wrinkled capsule with muddy red appearance on cut section
- Microscopically, complete destruction of hepatocytes with preserved portal tracts with little to no inflammation.

Acute hepatitis

- Ballooning degeneration of hepatocytes.
- Cholestasis
- Lymphocytic infiltration around degenerating hepatocytes
- Bridging necrosis—between portal to portal, portal to central and central to central of adjacent hepatic lobules
- Kupffer cell hypertrophy and hyperplasia
- Portal inflammation
- Interface hepatitis—Spillover of inflammatory cells from portal tract into adjacent parenchyma causing necrosis of periportal hepatocytes.

VIRAL HEPATITIS (contd.)

Specific types

Viral hepatitis A

- It is caused by hepatitis A virus (HAV) which is a small, non-enveloped single stranded RNA Picornavirus
- It spreads by feco-oral route
- Incubation period is 15–40 days
- It is a transient infection and no carrier state or chronic hepatitis seen
- There is no malignant transformation noted.

Viral hepatitis B

- It is caused by hepatitis B virus (HBV) which is an enveloped double stranded DNA virus of Hepadnavirus family
- The virion is called *Dane particle*
- It spreads by parenteral route or close physical contact
- Incubation period is 30–180 days
- Carrier state is seen in up to 1% of individuals
- Transformation to chronic hepatitis occur in 5–10% of individuals
- It can undergo malignant transformation to hepatocellular carcinoma.

Serological markers of viral hepatitis A

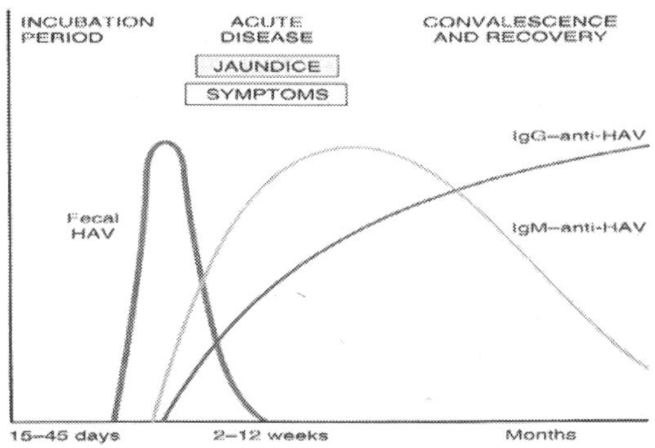

Serological markers of chronic viral hepatitis B

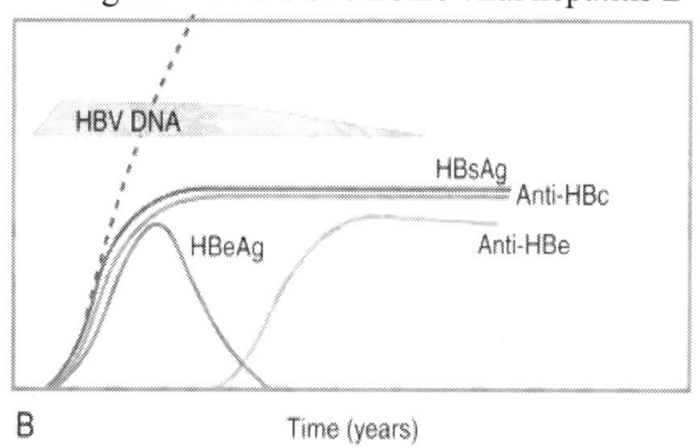

Serological markers of acute viral hepatitis B

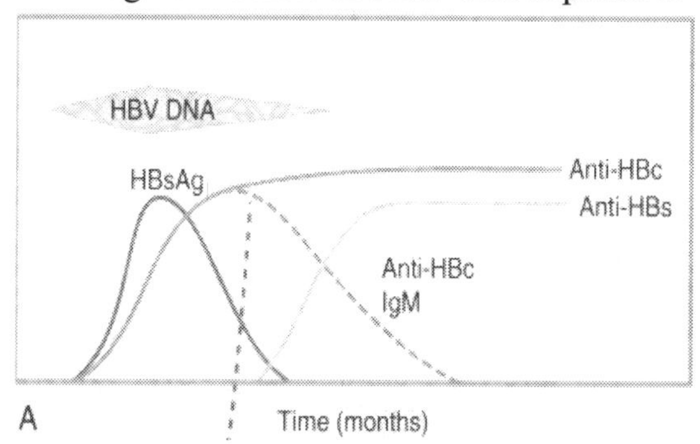

VIRAL HEPATITIS (contd.) → **Specific types (contd.)**

Viral hepatitis C

- It is caused by hepatitis C virus (HCV) which is an enveloped short stranded RNA virus
- Mode of transmission is parenteral and close physical contact
- Incubation period is 30–50 days
- Carrier state – seen in intravenous drug abusers and repeated blood transfused patients
- Chronic hepatitis is seen in 30–45% cases.
- Transformation to hepatocellular carcinoma is noted.

Serological markers of chronic viral hepatitis C

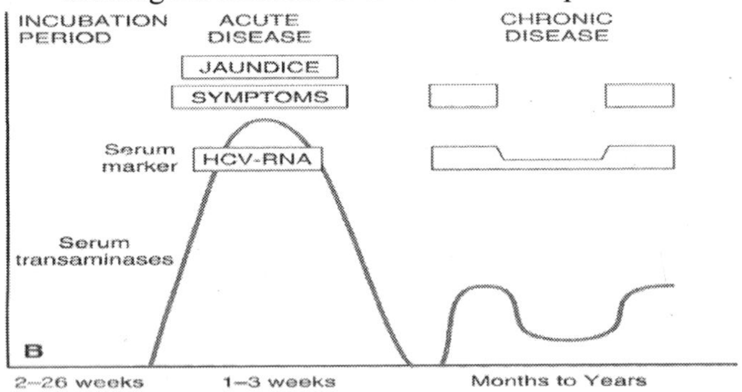

Serological markers of acute viral hepatitis C

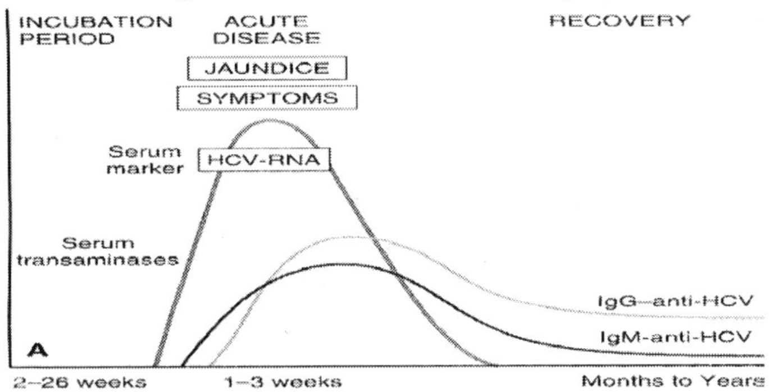

HEPATOCELLULAR CARCINOMA (HCC)

Definition: It is the most common malignant tumor of the hepatocytes of liver.

- M : F ratio is 1.5–3:1
- Age group is 20–40 yrs (in high hepatitis B viral infection communities) and >60 years (in low hepatitis B viral infection communities).

Tumor markers: Serum α-fetoprotein is elevated in two-thirds of patients with HCC.

Morphology

Gross morphology (Image R)

- It appears grossly as:
  - Unifocal
  - Multifocal
  - Diffusely infiltrative cancer
- Tumor is slightly paler than normal liver.

Microscopy (Fig. 39)

- They range from well-differentiated to anaplastic undifferentiated lesion
- Tumor cells are arranged in trabeculae or pseudoglandular pattern and have abundant eosinophilic cytoplasm and pleomorphic hyperchromatic nuclei
- Fibrolamellar variant—It occurs in younger age group, not associated with HBV infection and shows strong desmoplasia.

Etiopathogenesis

- Hepatitis B viral infection:
  - 85% cases occur in countries with high incidence of chronic viral hepatitis B infection
  - Chronic HBV infection increases the risk of HCC by 200 times
  - Risk of hepatocellular carcinoma is 4 times in patients who are positive for both HBs and HBe antigens as compared to those who are positive for HBs antigen only.
- Hepatitis C viral infection:
  - HCV is a more common cause of HCC in countries with low prevalence of HBV infection
  - Risk of HCC in patients with both HBV and HCV infection is 3 times higher than either of them alone.
- Dietary factors:
  - Alcoholic cirrhosis predisposes to HCC
  - Intake of foods containing aflatoxin B increases the risk of HCC by 3 times
  - Patients with hemochromatosis and α_1-antitrypsin deficiency have 10% higher risk of developing HCC.

CHOLELITHIASIS

Definition: It is defined as the presence of stones within the lumen of gallbladder or extrahepatic biliary tree.

Types

Cholesterol stones
They comprise 70–80% of gall stones.

Morphology
- Cholesterol stones are pale yellow, round to ovoid with finely granular, hard surface.
- Cholesterol ranges from 100–50% in them.
- Pure cholesterol stones are radiolucent.

Pigment stones: They comprise 20% of the gallstones.

Morphology: They are classified into two types.

Brown pigment stones:
- They are found in infected gallbladder bile
- They contain calcium salt of unconjugated bilirubin, palmitate, stearate and mucin glycoprotein
- They are radiolucent.

Black pigment stones (Image S)
- They are formed in sterile gallbladder bile
- They contain oxidized polymers of calcium salts of unconjugated bilirubin, calcium carbonate, mucin and calcium phosphate
- They are up to 15 cm in size, multiple and crumble on touch
- They are moulded and have spicules
- They are radio-opaque.

Etiology
- Risk factors includes:
  - Asian population
  - Patients with chronic hemolytic diseases
  - Biliary tract infection by *E. coli, Ascaris lumbricoides* or liver fluke
  - Gastrointestinal disorders, e.g. Crohn disease, cystic fibrosis.

Pathogenesis

Cholesterol stones
- Formation of cholesterol stones is a multifactorial process depending on following factors:
  - Supersaturation of cholesterol in bile
  - Gallbladder hypomotility
  - Extensive secretion of mucous from gall-bladder mucosa
  - Accelarated nucleation of cholesterol crystals.

Pigment stones
- Black pigment stone is formed in chronic hemolytic conditions, e.g. sickle cell anemia, thalassemia due to increased formation of bilirubin
- Brown pigment stone is found in association with bacterial or parasitic cholangitis; enzymes released by them convert conjugated bilirubin to unconjugated bilirubin leading to stone formation.

PANCREATITIS

Acute pancreatitis

Definition: It is defined as an inflammatory condition of exocrine pancreas resulting from injury to acini.

Complications
- Shock
- Acute renal failure
- Disseminated intravascular coagulation
- Pancreatic abscess
- Pancreatic pseudocyst

Etiology
- Alcohol
- Hypercalcemia
- Hyperlipoproteinemia
- Trauma
- Gallstones
- Iatrogenic
- Shock
- Mumps
- Coxsackievirus infection.

Morphology
- The pancreas exhibits red black areas of hemorrhage with foci of yellow white, chalky fat necrosis.
- Microscopically, acinar cell necrosis, acute inflammatory infiltrate and foci showing necrotic fat cells are seen.

Pathogenesis
- Activation of trypsinogen to trypsin is important trigger for acute pancreatitis
- Trypsin activates other enzyme like elestase, phospholipase and kallikrein
- Activation of pancreatic enzymes occur by 3 pathways:
  - Acinar cell injury
  - Pancreatic duct obstruction
  - Defective intracellular transport of proenzymes within acinar cells.

Chronic pancreatitis

Etiology: Causes are same for both acute and chronic pancreatitis.

Complications
- Pseudocyst
- Duct obstruction
- Steatorrhea
- Secondary diabetes.

Pathogenesis: Same as for acute pancreatitis.

Morphology
- Grossly, pancreas is firm with loss of lobular appearance; pancreatic ducts are dilated with luminal obstruction
- Microscopically, parenchymal fibrosis, reduction in exocrine elements, duct dilatation and lymphohistiocytic infiltrate in stroma is noted.

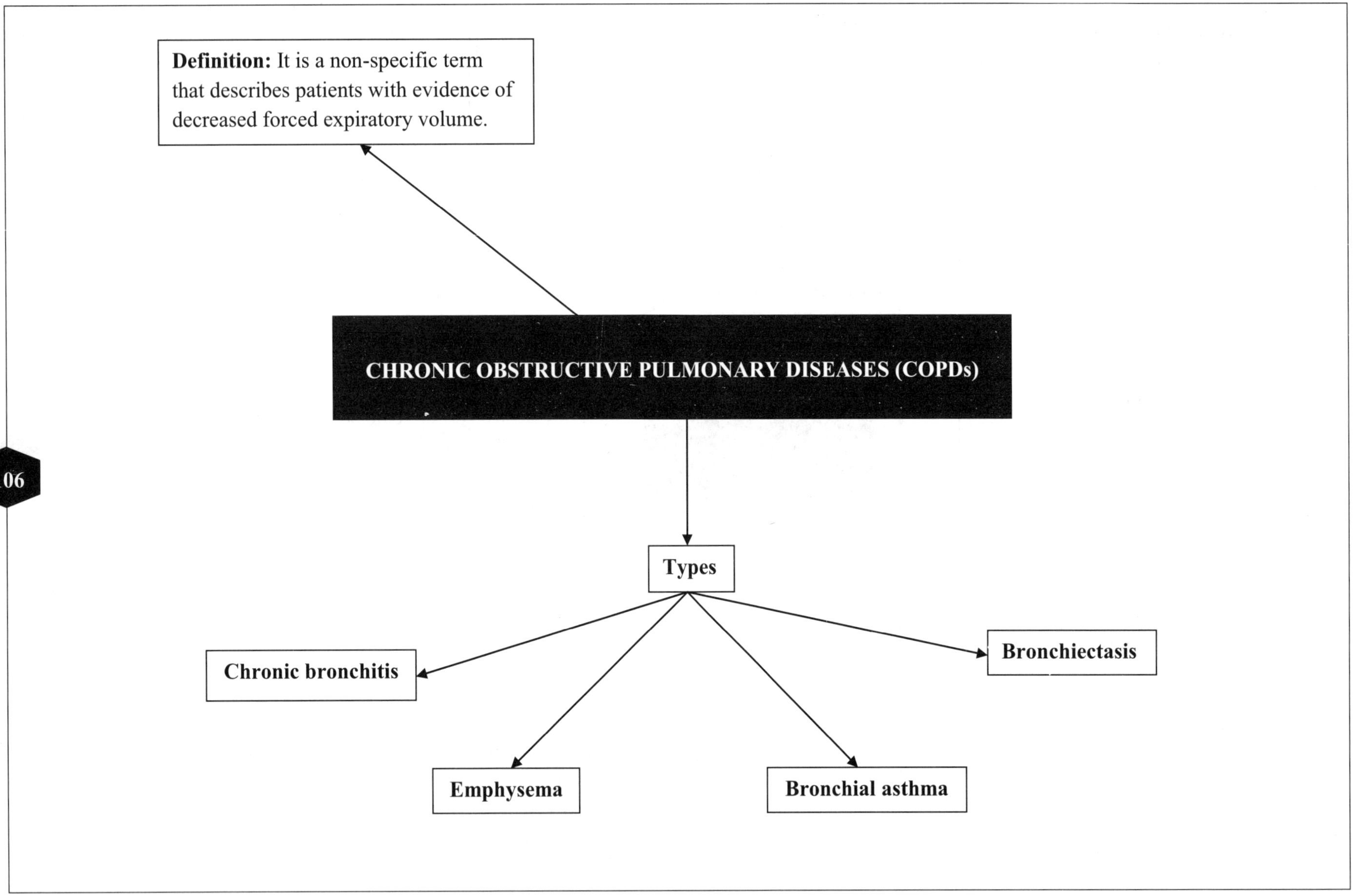
Definition: It is a non-specific term that describes patients with evidence of decreased forced expiratory volume.
CHRONIC OBSTRUCTIVE PULMONARY DISEASES (COPDs)
Types
Chronic bronchitis
Emphysema
Bronchial asthma
Bronchiectasis

CHRONIC BRONCHITIS

Definition: It is defined as persistent cough with sputum production in a patient for three months in two consecutive years without any discernible cause.

Etiopathogenesis

- 90% of causes occur in cigarette smokers
- 5–10% cases occur due to atmospheric pollutants
- Due to chronic irritation, there is hypersecretion of mucous with goblet cell hyperplasia
- Acute exacerbation occurs due to secondary bacterial and viral infections.

Morphology

Microscopy

- There is hyperplasia and hypertrophy of mucous glands associated with dense lymphocytic infiltrate in surrounding stroma
- There is squamous metaplasia noted in the bronchial epithelium
- Reid index is increased from normal value of 0.4 and it is defined as the measure of vertical thickness of mucous gland layer to the thickness of bronchial wall up to the perichondrium.

Gross morphology

- There is swelling, hyperemia and edema of bronchiolar mucous membranes
- There is occlusion of lumen of involved bronchiole by pus and mucous.

EMPHYSEMA

Definition: It is a chronic lung disease characterized by abnormal permanent enlargement of airspaces distal to terminal bronchioles accompanied by destruction of their walls without obvious fibrosis.

Etiopathogenesis

- Cigarette smoking is the major cause of emphysema
- The pathogenesis is best explained by protease-antiprotease theory
- α_1-antitrypsin is an antiprotease enzyme present in the serum and interstitial tissue
- In smokers, neutrophils are sequested into lung alveoli where they release elastase along with interleukin 8, leukotriene B_4 and tumor necrosis factor
- The imbalance between neutrophil elastase and α_1-antitrypsin results in dilatation of lung alveoli and later, emphysema
- Tobacco smoke releases reactive oxygen species that deplete the antioxidants present in the lung alveoli.

Morphology

Microscopy (Fig. 41)

- There are abnormally large alveoli separated by thin fibrous septae seen.

Gross morphology

- The lungs are voluminous especially in panacinar emphysema
- In distal acinar emphysema, large subpleural blebs are seen.

Types

Centriacinar emphysema

- The central or proximal part of acini are involved sparing the distal alveoli
- It is more common in upper lobes
- It is most commonly seen in smokers.

Irregular emphysema

- The acinus is irregularly involved.

Distal acinar emphysema

- It is also known as *paraseptal emphysema*
- It is more common in upper half of lung adjacent to pleura.

Panacinar emphysema

- In this type, the acini are uniformly enlarged from the level of respiratory bronchiole to terminal blind alveoli
- It is more common in lower zones and anterior margin of lung
- It is seen in patients with α_1-antitrypsin deficiency.

BRONCHIECTASIS

Definition: It is a condition characterized by permanent dilatation of bronchi and bronchioles cause by destruction of elastic and muscular tissue secondary to chronic necrotizing infections.

Etiology

- Bronchiectasis develops in the following conditions:
  - Bacterial pneumonia
  - Viral pneumonia
  - Fungal pneumonia
  - Bronchial obstruction secondary to tumors, foreign bodies
  - Autoimmune diseases like rheumatoid arthritis, inflammatory bowel disease
  - Cystic fibrosis
  - Kartegener syndrome
  - Intralobar lung sequestration.

Pathogenesis

- Obstruction and infection are influences associated with bronchiectasis
- Obstruction of the airway leads to repeated infections that cause damage to the bronchial and bronchiolar walls leading to dilatation.

Morphology

Microscopy (Fig. 40)

- There is intense inflammatory infiltrate seen within the walls of bronchi and bronchioles
- The lining epithelium may show ulceration or pseudostratification of lining cell or squamous metaplasia of the lining epithelium
- In chronic cases, bronchial and peribronchial fibrosis is seen.

Gross morphology (Image T)

- It affects the lower lobes bilaterally more so on the right side
- Airways are dilated sometimes up to 3–4 times normal
- Grossly, they are classified as:
  - Saccular
  - Fusiform
  - Cylindrical
- Cut surface of the lung shows dilated bronchial cysts filled with mucopurulent secretions.

BRONCHIAL ASTHMA

Definition: It is a chronic inflammatory disorder of the airways that causes recurrent episodes of wheezing, breathlessness, chest tightness and cough associated with bronchospasm in response to a variety of stimuli.

Types: Based on type of antigen, asthma is classified into:

- *Extrinsic asthma*: It is initiated by type I hypersensitivity reaction in response to external antigen
- *Intrinsic asthma*: It is initiated by non-immune mechanisms such as aspirin ingestion, pulmonary infections, stress and exercise.

Pathogenesis

- Etiological factors of asthma are predisposition to type I hypersensitivity, acute and chronic airway inflammation as well as bronchial hyper responsiveness
- TH_2 helper CD4 + T-cells secrete interleukins 3 and 5 which recruit eosinophils at the site as wells as interleukin-4 which activate B-cells to produce IgE antibodies and mast cells on presentation of antigen by antigen presenting cells to T-lymphocyte
- The mast cells and eosinophils release mediators that cause increased vascular permeability and smooth muscle contraction.

Morphology

Microscopy

- The mucous plugs are composed of whorls of epithelial cells enmeshed with mucous and are known as *Curschmann spirals*
- There is thickening of bronchial epithelial basement membrane
- There is eosinophil and mast cell infiltrate in bronchial wall.

Gross morphology

- The lungs are overdistended due to hyperinflation
- There is occlusion of bronchus and bronchioles by mucous plugs.

PNEUMOCONIOSIS

Definition: It is defined as non-neoplastic lung reaction to occupational exposure of mineral dusts.

Pathogenesis

- Development of pneumoconiosis depends on:
  - Amount of dust retained in respiratory tract
  - Size and shape of particle
  - Solubility of particle
  - Capacity of dust particle to induce fibrosis
- The most dangerous particles are 1–5 μm in diameter that reach up to the alveoli.

Various types of pneumoconiosis

Dusts	-	Disease
Coal dust	-	Anthracosis
Silica dust	-	Silicosis
Asbestos	-	Asbestosis
Beryllium	-	Berylliosis
Moldy hay	-	Farmer's lung
Cotton	-	Byssinosis

Coal workers pneumoconiosis (CWP)

- Exposure to coal dust leads to development of spectrum of lung finding which include:
  - Asymptomatic anthracosis: In this, the patient is asymptomatic and pulmonary lesion shows carbon laden interstitial macrophages
  - Simple coal workers pneumoconiosis– It is characterized by coal macules 1–2 mm in diameter to slightly larger coal nodules. The macules are composed of coal dust laden macrophages whereas nodules are composed of macrophages with variable amount of collagen. They predominantly involve upper lobe and upper portion of lower lobe
  - Complicated CWP – In this, the lesion is black and varies from 2–10 cm in size, multiple with lesion containing collagen and coal dust.

PNEUMOCONIOSIS (contd.)

Asbestosis

Definition

- It refers to diffuse interstitial fibrosis in lung that results from inhalation of asbestos fibres.

Pathogenesis

- Asbestos fibres are long (up to 100 μm) and thin (0.5–1 μm) which enter into the intestinal space of lung and induce fibrosing inflammation
- Chronic exposure may lead to tumor formation.

Morphology

- Asbestos exposure induces a variety of lesions which include:
    - Benign pleural effusion
    - Pleural plaques
    - Diffuse pleural fibrosis
    - Pulmonary interstitial fibrosis
    - In lung; along with fibrosis, asbestos bodies are seen which appear as golden brown, fusiform or beaded rods with translucent centre
    - Long-standing exposure may lead to development of lung cancers and pleural as well as peritoneal mesotheliomas.

LUNG ABSCESS

Definition: It is a localized accumulation of pus accompanied by destruction of pulmonary parenchyma including alveoli, airways and blood vessels.

Etiopathogenesis

- Conditions predisposing to lung abscess include:
  - Alcohol intake
  - Drug overdose
  - Epileptics
  - Oropharnyngeal surgical operation
  - Sinobronchial infections
  - Necrotizing pneumonias
  - Bronchial obstruction
  - Infected pulmonary emboli
  - Trauma
- Arobic and anarobic bacteria are common causative organisms of lung abscess.

Morphology

Microscopy

- Abscess contains suppurative debris composed of live and dead neutrophils, fibrin and coagulative necrosis.

Gross morphology

- They vary in size from few millimetre to multiple centimetre
- They are single to multiple; more common one right side
- Abscess due to aspiration are single
- Pneumonic abscesses are multiple, diffuse and basal.

PNEUMONIA

Definition: It is defined as infection of a lobe of lung or entire lung.

Types
- Community acquired acute pneumonia
- Community acquired atypical pneumonia
- Nosocomial pneumonia
- Aspiration pneumonia
- Chronic pneumonia
- Pneumonia in immunocompromised patients.

Etiopathogenesis
- It develops due to impairment of respiratory defense mechanism which include:
  - Inhibition of cough reflex
  - Pulmonary congestion and edema
  - Impairment of mucociliary apparatus
  - Inhibition of phagocytic action of alveolar macrophages
  - Accumulation of secretions
- Pneumonia is caused by bacteria, virus, fungus, parasites and *Mycoplasma.*

Morphology

Gross morphology
- Grossly, pneumonias are of two types:
  - *Lobar pneumonia*: There is involvement of a large portion of a lobe or entire lobe
  - *Bronchopneumonia*: There are multiple, patchy areas of consolidation seen involving multiple lobes of both lungs.

Microscopy
- Lobar pneumonia has four stages:
  - *Stage of congestion*: There is vascular congestion with intra-alveolar fluid and neutrophils
  - *Stage of red hepatization*: There is dense neutrophilic infiltration of alveoli with fibrin deposition
  - *Stage of grey hepatization*: Red cells degenerate and form hemosiderin to give rise to grey colour of lung tissue
  - *Stage of resolution*: Macrophages phagocytose necrotic debris
- In bronchopneumonia, there are multiple foci of neutrophils with necrotic debris seen.

BRONCHOGENIC CARCINOMA

Definition: It is the most common cancer in lung which develops secondary to carcinogenic effects of cigarette smoke.

Classification: Based on major histological pattern, they are of 4 types:
- Small cell carcinoma
- Squamous cell carcinoma
- Adenocarcinoma
- Large cell carcinoma.

Etiology: Major risk factors causing lung carcinoma are:
- *Tobacco smoking*
  - Heavy cigarette smokers have 10–60 times higher risk
  - Cigar and pipe smokers have lesser risk
  - Carcinogens in smoke are benzopyrene, phenol derivatives, $carbon^{14}$, $polonium^{210}$ etc.
- *Occupational exposure*
  - Exposure to asbestos increases risk 5–10 times
  - Asbestos workers who smoke have 90 times higher risk
  - Atomic bomb survivors exposed to radiation have high risk
- *Air pollution*
  - Radon exposure increases risk.

Pathogenesis
- In small cell carcinomas, mutations in c-MYC and RB genes occur
- In non-small cell carcinomas, mutation in RAS and p16 genes is noted.

Morphology

Microscopy
- *Squamous cell carcinoma*
  - Occur in smoker males and is central in location
  - Tumor cells arranged in solid sheets and small clusters with variable amount of keratinization
- *Adenocarcinoma*
  - Seen in non-smokers and women
  - They are peripheral in location
  - Tumor cells are arranged in papillae, acini and solid patterns with variable amount of mucin
- *Large cell carcinoma*
  - They are undifferentiated malignant tumors
  - Tumor cells are large with moderate cytoplasm and large nucleus with prominent nucleoli
- *Small cell carcinoma*
  - Highly malignant tumor strongly associated with smoking
  - Tumor cells are round oval and spindle shaped with scant cytoplasm, ill-defined cell margins and nucleus with salt and pepper chromatin.

Gross morphology (Image U)
- Grossly, bronchogenic carcinomas present as cauliflower like grey white hard mass with areas of necrosis and hemorrhage
- Extension into pleura is seen in late stages
- Lymphatic metastasis to tracheal, bronchial and mediastinal lymph nodes noted
- Metastasis occurs to liver, brain and bone.

TESTICULAR TUMORS

SEMINOMA

- They are most common testicular cancer accounting for 40–50% of all germ cell tumors of testis
- Age—They are seen majorly in 30–40 years age group.

Subtypes

- Seminoma with syncytiotrophoblastic giant cells
- Anaplastic seminoma
- Spermatocytic seminoma

Morphology

- Grossly, they are large solid, greyish, rubbery firm bosselated mass **(Image V)**
- Microscopically, they present as sheets of monomorphic cells separated by delicate fibrous septae
- The tumor cells are round to polyhedral with distinct cell membrane, clear or watery cytoplasm and a large central nucleus with 1–2 prominent nucleoli
- The fibrous septae show T-lymphocytes and rarely granuloma.

Etiology: Risk factors for testicular tumors include:

- *Cryptorchidism*: Higher the location of undescended testis, greater is the risk of developing cancer.
- *Testicular dysgenesis*: Patients with Klinefelter's syndrome and testicular ferminization syndrome harbor the risk of development of germ cell tumors
- *i (12p)*: Isochromosome of short arm of chromosome 12 is found in all germ cell tumors.

Classification

- Germ cell tumors (90%)
  - Seminoma (40–50%)
  - Non-seminomatous germ cell tumors
    - Embryonal carcinoma
    - Teratoma
    - Yolk sac tumor
    - Choriocarcinoma
- Sex cord stromal tumors (5%)
  - Leydig cell tumor
  - Sertoli cell tumor
- Metastatic tumors (5%)

Tumor markers

- α-fetoprotein (AFP) is elevated in yolk sac tumors
- Human chorionic gonadotrophin (hCG) is elevated in choriocarcinoma
- Placental alkaline phosphatase (PLAP) is elevated in seminoma
- Lactate dehydrogenase (LDH) is a non-specific marker of testicular tumors and indicates tumor burden.

- Tumors of testis account for <1% of all malignancies in adults
- 90% of the tumors are germ cell tumors.

Pathogenesis

- Majority of testicular tumors originate from intratubular germ cell neoplasia (ITGCN)
- Neoplastic germinal cells differentiate towards gonadal lines to give rise to seminoma
- If neoplastic germinal cells transform into totipotential cell line, it gives rise to non-seminomatous germ cell tumors
- If totipotential cells stay undifferentiated, they form embryonal carcinoma
- Totipotential cells differentiate along extraembryonic line to give rise to yolk sac tumor or choriocarcinoma.

BENIGN PROSTATIC HYPERPLASIA (BPH)

Definition: It is a common disorder characterized clinically by enlargement of the gland and obstruction to the flow of urine through the bladder outlet and pathologically by proliferation of glands and stroma.

Pathogenesis

- Dihydrotestosterone (DHT) is a metabolite of testosterone synthesized by the action of enzyme 5α-reductase located in stromal cells on testosterone
- DHT binds with nuclear androgen receptor and causes signal transcription of growth factors which are mitogenic to epithelial and stromal cells
- DHT is 10 times more potent then testosterone in androgen receptor binding and produce hyperplasia.

Morphology

Gross morphology (Image W)

- Origin of BPH occurs from transitional zone of prostate
- Grossly, the prostate is enlarged to form multiple nodules
- The nodules with fibromuscular elements are pale grey
- The nodules with glandular element are yellow pink.

Microscopy (Fig. 42)

- Microscopically, nodularity is due to glandular and fibromuscular proliferation
- Glands are small to large cystically dilated lined by inner columnar and outer cuboidal epithelium lying on intact basement membrane
- Foci of infarction and squamous metaplasia are also noted.

PROSTATIC CARCINOMA

- It is the most common cancer in men and second most common cause of death
- Adenocarcinoma is the most common type.

Etiology

- Age—seen in >50 years old males; risk increases with age
- Diet—Excess intake of dietary fat increases risk; diet rich in antioxidants reduces the risk
- Testosterone also plays a significant role in its development
- Family history—Men with one first degree relative have two times and two first degree relatives with prostatic carcinoma have 5-fold increased risk.

Grading and prognosis

- Gleason score is used to grade prostate adenocarcinomas and a total score of 10 is given
- Score of 2–4 represents well-differentiated adenocarcinoma and has good prognosis
- Score of 5–7 represents moderately differentiated adenocarcinoma
- Score of >7 represents poorly differentiated adenocarcinoma and indicates poor prognosis.

Pathogenesis

- Androgens play a role in its causation
- Amplification of androgen receptor gene increases sensitivity of prostatic epithelium to testosterone and cause cancerogenesis
- Genetic damage to gene located on 1q chromosome leads to increased risk of familial prostatic carcinoma.

Tumor markers

- Prostate specific antigen (PSA):
  - It is an enzyme which functions to cleave and liquefy semen after ejaculation
  - It is secreted from prostatic epithelium
  - Serum PSA levels of 4 ng/ml is cut-off point between normal and abnormal
  - Serum PSA level of 4–10 ng/ml indicate grey zone, i.e. the condition can be malignant or benign
  - Serum PSA level of >10 ng/ml indicate prostate cancer in 80% cases.

Morphology (Fig. 43)

- Site of origin—peripheral zone of prostate
- Grossly, it is invisible within the gland; only firm to cut
- Microscopically, cancer glands are small irregular and lack branching or papillae; the outer basal layer is absent and tumor cells have pleomorphic nuclei
- Metastasis occurs locally to seminal vesicle or bladder and hematogenously into the axial skeleton.

CYSTIC RENAL DISEASES

Definition: They are a group of hereditary, developmental and non-hereditary, acquired disorders characterized by cyst formations within the renal parenchyma.

Classification
- Cystic renal dysplasia
- Polycystic kidney disease
- Medullary sponge kidney
- Nephronophthisis
- Acquired cystic disease
- Simple renal cysts
- Glomerular cysts.

Polycystic kidney disease

Autosomal recessive (Infantile) polycystic kidney disease
- It is a congenital renal disease characterized by cystic transformation of collecting ducts.

Gross morphology
- External surface of kidney is smooth
- There is bilateral involvement of the kidney.

Associated complications
- Congenital hepatic fibrosis.

Microscopy
- The cysts are fusiform dilatations of cortical and medullary collecting ducts lined by cuboidal epithelium.

Pathogenesis
- It is caused by mutation in PKHD 1 gene located on chromosome 6.

Autosomal dominant (adult) polycystic kidney disease
- It is the most common of a group of congenital diseases that are characterized by numerous cysts within renal parenchyma.

Microscopy
- The cysts arise from any part of nephron from glomerulus upto the collecting tubules
- Normal renal parenchyma is seen in between the cysts
- The lining of the cysts is variable depending upon the site of origin.

Associated complications
- Cysts in liver, pancreas and spleen.
- Subarachnoid hemorrhage secondary to rupture of berry aneurysms in circle of Willis.

Pathogenesis
- 85% of autosomal dominant polycystic kidney disease are caused by mutations in PKD1 gene, 15% by mutation in PKD2 gene and <1% by mutation in PKD3 gene.

Gross pathology (Image X)
- Bilateral markedly enlarged kidneys.
- External surface distorted by multiple cysts.
- The cysts are 0.5–5 cm in diameter and is filled with straw colored fluid.

NEPHROTIC SYNDROME

Definition: It is a clinical syndrome characterized by heavy proteinuria (>3.5g/24 hours), hypoalbuminemia, edema, hyperlipidemia and lipiduria.

Pathophysiology

Glomerular injury
↓
Increased permeability of glomerular capillaries to protein
↓
Proteinuria
↓
Decreased serum protein
↓ (leads to two branches)

- Decreased plasma oncotic pressure
  - → Plasma escape in tissues → Edema
  - → Decreased plasma volume → Decreased glomerular filtration rate → Fluid retention → Edema
- Compensatory synthesis of lipoprotenis and other proteins from liver → Hyperlipidemia

Causes

Secondary causes

- Diabetes mellitus
- SLE
- Amyloidosis
- Infections—Malaria, syphilis, hepatitis B and C, AIDS
- Drugs—Non-steroidal anti-inflammatory drugs
- Malignancies—Carcinoma, lymphoma.

NEPHROTIC SYNDROME (contd.)

Causes (contd.)

Primary causes
- Minimal change disease.
- Membranous glomerulopathy.
- Focal segmental glomerulosclerosis.
- Membranoproliferative glomerulonephritis.

Membranous glomerulopathy
- It is the most common cause of nephrotic syndrome in adults characterized by diffuse thickening of glomerular capillary wall and accumulation of electron dense immunoglobulin deposits along the subepithelial side of the basement membrane.

Morphology
- Glomeruli are slightly enlarged but normocellular
- Glomerular capillary walls are normal or thickened
- On silver stains, spikes are seen on epithelial surface of basement membrane
- In advanced lesions, the glomerular capillary is obliterated leading to sclerosis.

Pathogenesis
- It is a chronic immune complex mediated disease
- The antibodies are formed against the podocytes
- The immune complex formed are shed into subepithelial zone where they bind to produce manifestations.

Minimal change nephropathy (Lipoid nephrosis)
- It is the most common cause of nephrotic syndrome in children characterized by diffuse effacetment of foot processes of epithelial cells in glomeruli that appear normal on light microscopy.

Morphology
- Grossly, kidney is absolutely normal
- On light microscopy, the glomeruli are normal
- On electron mircoscopy, there is diffuse effacement of the foot processes of visceral epithelial cells.

Pathogenesis
- Cause is unknown
- It is most probably due to immune mediated injury suggested by remission on corticosteroid therapy, its association with Hodgkin lymphoma and other T-cell lymphomas.

NEPHRITIC SYNDROME

Definition: It is a clinical syndrome characterized by hematuria, variable degree of proteinuria and decreased glomerular filtration rate resulting in elevated levels of blood urea nitrogen, serum creatinine, oliguria, salt and water retention, edema and hypertension.

Causes

Secondary causes

- Diabetes mellitus
- SLE
- Amyloidosis
- Inections
- Drugs—Non-steroidal anti-inflammatory drugs, pencillamine
- Malignancies—carcinoma, lymphoma.

Pathogenesis

- Glomerulonephritis is caused by immunological mechanisms
- Both antibody and cell-mediated immunity plays a role
- 3 mechanism of antibody induced inflammation are incriminated in majority of areas which include:
  - *In situ* immune complex formation
  - Deposition of circulating immune complexes
  - Anti-neutrophil cytoplasmic antibody.

NEPHRITIC SYNDROME (contd.)

Causes (contd.)

Primary causes: The causes are in decreasing order of frequency
- Crescentic glomerulonephritis (RPGN)
- Acute post-streptococcal glomerulonephritis (PSGN)
- Membranoproliferative glomerulonephritis (MPGN)
- Focal segmental glomerulosclerosis (FSGS)
- Membranous glomerulonephritis (MGN)

Rapidly progressive (crescentic) glomerulonephritis
- It is a syndrome associated with severe glomerular injury characterized by presence of crescents in most of the glomeruli.

Classification and pathogenesis
It is classified into three types:
- Type I RPGN (Anti-GBM antibody type)
  - Idiopathic
  - Goodpasture syndrome
- Type II RPGN (Immune complex mediated)
  - Idiopathic
  - Post-infections
  - SLE
  - Henoch-Schonlein purpura
- Type III RPGN (Pauci-immune)
  - ANCA associated
  - Wegener granulomatosis
  - Polyarteritis nodosa.

Morphology
- Grossly, kidneys are enlarged and pale with petechial hemorrhages on cortical surface
- Microscopically, crescents are formed by proliferation of parietal cells and migration of monocytes and macrophages in urinary space
- Glomeruli show focal necrosis, diffuse or focal endothelial and mesangial proliferation.

Membranoproliferative glomerulonephritis
- It is a type of glomerulonephritis characterized by alterations in the basement membrane, glomerular proliferation and infiltration by leukocytes
- It is also called *mesangiocapillary glomerulonephritis*.

Classification

Secondary MPGN: It arises in following conditions:
- Autoimmune diseases – SLE, hepatitis B, hepatitis C.
- α_1-antitrypsin deficiency.
- Cancers – CLL, lymphoma.

Primary or idiopathic MPGN
- They are of two types based on ultrastructural features: Type I and Type II
- Microscopically, glomeruli are large and hypercellular.
- There is mesangial and capillary endothelial cell hypercellularity seen.
- Glomerular capillary wall shows tram track appearance.

- Type I MPGN
  - Presence of subendothelial electron dense deposits
  - Immunoflourescence show C3 and IgG
- Type II MPGN
  - There is dense deposition of C3 in glomerular basement (GBM) membrane with absence of IgG.

SYSTEMIC DISEASES WITH GLOMERULONEPHRITIS

Diabetic nephropathy

- It is seen in 30–45% cases of diabetes mellitus.
- The lesions seen in diabetes mellitus are:
  - Non-nephrotic proteinuria
  - Nephrotic syndrome
  - Chronic renal failure
  - Papillary necrosis
  - Arteriosclerosis.

Pathogenesis

- Advanced glycosylated end products are produced causing glomerulopathy
- Hyperglycemia in diabetics cause increased synthesis of collagen type II and decreased synthesis of heparan sulfate in glomerular basement membrane (GBM).

Morphology

- Glomerular enlargement, GBM thickening and mesangial hypercellularity is the earliest lesion
- Diffuse glomerulosclerosis – diffuse thickening of GBM and mesangial matrix expansion
- Nodular glomerulosclerosis—It is also called *Kimmelstiel-Wilson disease*; there are PAS positive nodules seen in the periphery of glomerulus.

Systemic lupus erythematosus nephritis

- The lesions in SLE are due to immune complex deposition in the glomeruli
- The glomerular lesions are classified into five groups:
  - Minimal lesion (Type I)
  - Mesangial lupus glomerulonephritis (Type II)
  - Focal proliferative glomerulonephritis (Type III)
  - Diffuse proliferative glomerulonephritis (Type IV)
  - Membranous glomerulonephritis (Type V)

CHRONIC PYELONEPHRITIS

Definition: It is a chronic renal disease characterized by infection of renal tubules, interstitium and renal pelvis.

Etiology

The causative agents include:

- *E. coli*
- *Klebsiella*
- *Proteus*
- *Staphylococcus*
- *Streptococcus fecalis*
- *Cytomegalovirus*
- *Adenovirus*

The predisposing conditions are:

- Urinary tract obstruction
- Catheterization
- Vesicoureteral reflux
- Pregnancy
- Diabetes mellitus
- Immunodeficiency diseases.

Pathogenesis

- It is most commonly caused by ascending infection.
- Steps in pathogenesis are:

Colonization of distal urethra by microbes

↓

They gain access from urethra to urinary bladder

↓

Organism multiply in bladder

↓

Vesioureteral reflux of urine from urinary bladder to renal pelvis and calyces due to either incompetence of urethrovesical valve or due to obstruction.

Morphology

- Grossly, there is irregular scarring seen in one or both kidneys
- There is a corticomedullary scar seen overlying a dilated calyx
- Microscopically, there is periglomerular fibrosis, tubular atrophy, thyroidization of tubules and chronic interstitial inflammation with or without fibrosis seen. **(Fig. 44)**

HYPERTENSIVE NEPHROPATHY

Benign nephrosclerosis: It is defined as a disease associated with renal artery and arteriolar sclerosis secondary to hypertension.

Morphology

- Grossly, the kidneys are smaller than normal with bilateral involvement; the cortical surface is coarse and granular
- Microscopically, there is hyaline material deposition with thickening of renal arteriolar wall.

Malignant nephrosclerosis: It is defined as the renal pathological changes taking place in malignant hypertension.

Morphology

- Grossly, kidney may be enlarged or small with small hemorrhages on its cortical surface (Flea bitten kidney)
- Microscopically, there is fibrinoid necrosis seen in the interlobular arteries and arterioles associated with proliferation of smooth muscle cells with laying down of collagen (onion skin appearance).

RENAL STONES (NEPHROLITHIASIS)

Definition: Nephrolithiasis is stones within the collecting system of kidney and urolithiasis are stones within the collecting system of urinary tract

- Stones are unilateral in 80% patients
- Majority of them are formed in renal pelvis and calyces. **(Image Y)**

Types

Cystine stones

- They account for <1% of overall patients
- They are predominantly seen in children
- They occur exclusively in patients with hereditary cystinuria.

Uric acid stones

- They are seen in 5–10% patients
- They are associated with hyperuricemia
- They are radiolucent stones seen in patients with gout and post-cancer chemotherapy
- Morphologically, they are smooth and yellow with hard in consistency.

Calcium stones

- 70–75% of stones are calcium stones
- Majority of them are pure calcium oxalate with few are mixed with calcium phosphate
- Their formation is associated with hypercalcemia, hypercalciuria or hyperuricosuria
- They are radio-opaque
- Calcium oxalate stones are hard and dark coloured whereas calcium phosphate stones are soft and pale coloured.

Triple phosphate stones

- They are formed in urine post-infection with urea splitting bacteria e.g. *Proteus*
- They are composed of magnesium ammonium phosphate (struvite) and calcium phosphate (apatite)
- Infection stones fill the pelvis and calyces to produce stone casts called as *staghorn calculi*
- They are radio-opaque.

RENAL CELL CARCINOMA (RCC)

Definition: It is a malignant neoplasm of renal tubular or ductal epithelial cells

- It comprise 90% of all renal cancers
- Age group affected – 6th to 8th decade
- Sex – M : F : : 2 – 3 : 1

Etiology: The risk factor for renal cell carcinoma include:

- Cigarette smoking
- Obesity
- Hypertension
- Exposure to heavy metals and asbestos
- Estrogen therapy.

Pathogenesis

- 95% of renal cell carcinoma are sporadic; 5% are inherited
- Hereditary RCC occurs as three different syndromes:
    - Hereditary papillary RCC
    - Autosomal dominant clear cell RCC
    - von Hipple-Lindau syndrome.

Clinical features

- It is characterized by clinical triad of:
    - Hematuria
    - Flank pain
    - Palpable renal mass.

Morphology

Gross morphology (Image Z)

- Grossly, the tumor involves one of the poles of kidney
- Majority of RCC are seen in upper pole
- They occur as solitary or multiple grey white to bright yellow spherical masses with areas of necrosis and hemorrhage.

Microscopy: Based on microscopic features, they are classified into 4 groups:

- Clear cell RCC—They are characterized by sheets of clear cells with cytoplasmic vacuoles composed of glycogen and lipid; they comprise 80% of RCC **(Fig. 45)**
- Papillary RCC—These tumors arise from distal tubules and comprise 10 – 15% of RCC
- Chromophobe RCC—These tumors comprise 5% of RCC and are composed of tumor cells having abundant eosinophilic granular cytoplasm, well-defined cell margin and central round nucleus
- Collecting duct carcinoma—It comprises <1% of RCC.

WILMS TUMOR (NEPHROBLASTOMA)

Definition: It is the most common childhood abdominal malignant tumor

- It is usually unilateral; bilateral in 5–10% cases
- Also known as *nephroblastoma*
- Age group affected—2–5 years.

Etiology: Wilms tumors are sporadic or occur in association with:

- Denys-Drash syndrome
- WAGR syndrome
- Beckwith-Wiedemann syndrome

Clinical features

- Asymptomatic abdominal mass
- Abdominal pain
- Hematuria
- Hypertension
- Fever
- Urinary tract infection
- Varicocoele

Pathogenesis

- Mutation in WT1 tumor suppressor gene is associated with it.
- Mutation in IGF2 gene leading to its overexpression is associated with it.

Morphology

Gross morphology

- Grossly, the tumor is large, solitary, well-circumscribed; bilateral or multicentric in 5–10% cases
- Cut surface of tumor is soft, homogenous, grey tan in colour with foci of necrosis, hemorrhage and cyst formation.

Microscopy

- Tumor is triphasic, biphasic or rarely monophasic.
- Triphasic tumor show three components:
  - *Blastemal component*: Composed of small blue cells
  - *Epithelial component*: Composed of abortive tubules and glomeruli
  - *Stromal component*: Composed of fibrocytes in sheets
- Heterologous elements like neurogenic rests, smooth muscle, bone, cartilage, etc. may be seen.

UROTHELIAL CARCINOMA (TRANSITIONAL CELL CARCINOMA)

Specific features

- They are the most common urinary tract tumors
- They are seen in old age; median age is 65 yrs
- Males are affected thrice as common to females
- Majority of tumors are multifocal.

Etiology: Most important risk factors for urothelial carcinoma are:

- Cigarette smoking
- Industrial exposure to azodyes
- *Schistosoma hematobium* infection
- Radiotherapy for pelvic tumors
- Drugs like cyclophosphamide and NSAIDs.

Morphology

Microscopy (Fig. 46): Microscopically, urothelial carcinoma are of two types:

- *Low grade papillary urothelial carcinoma*: Cohesive tumor cells with minimal atypia; infrequent mitosis towards base; rarely invade deeper structures
- *High grade papillary urothelial carcinoma*: Dyscohesive tumor cells with frank anaplasia and frequent mitoses; deeply invasive and may be fatal.

Gross morphology

- The tumor has three variable gross appearances:
  - Exophytic (papillary or nodular)
  - Flat
  - Endophytic or infiltrative
- Papillary carcinoma arise from lateral wall near bladder base
- Flat carcinomas arise from lateral or posterior wall slightly away from the base of bladder.

Pathogenesis

- Deletion of 9p chromosome is the most common genetic damage seen in urothelial carcinoma affecting p16INK4a gene
- Other genetic abnormalities include del. 11p, 13p and 17p.

CARCINOMA CERVIX

Definition: It is the malignant tumor of cervix and is squamous cell carcinoma in 90–95% cases.

Etiology: The risk factors for carcinoma cervix include:

- Early age at first intercourse
- Multiple sexual partners
- Multiparous women
- Male partner with previous multiple sexual partners
- High-risk human papilloma virus, i.e. 16, 18, 31 and 33 subtypes infection
- Genital chlamydiasis.

Morphology

Microscopy

- The squamous cell carcinoma show three distinctive cellular patterns:
  - Large cell keratinizing type
  - Large cell non-keratinizing type
  - Small cell non-keratinizing type
- 80–90% of cervix carcinomas are squamous cell carcinoma whereas rest are adenocarcinoma or adenosquamous carcinomas.

Gross morphology (Image A1)

- It presents grossly as three different lesion:
  - Exophytic or fungating
  - Ulcerative lesion
  - Infiltrative lesion.

Pathogenesis

- High-risk HPV binds with nuclear DNA of squamous cells of cervix
- HPV E6 protein binds with p53 chromosome and inhibits cell death pathways
- HPV E 7 protein binds with Rb gene and upregulate cell cycle turnover
- These changes lead to cancer formation.

ADENOMYOSIS

Definition: It is defined as presence of endometrial glands or stroma or both in deeper portions of myometrium of uterus.

Morphology

Gross morphology: The myometrium shows small, red areas varying from 0.1 to 1 cm in size.

Microscopy: There are endometrial glands or stroma or both seen in between the fascicles of smooth muscle fibres with fibrosis surrounding the foci.

ENDOMETRIOSIS

Definition: It is defined as presence of endometrial glands or stroma or both in abnormal locations outside uterus.

Morphology

Gross morphology: The lesions of endometriosis vary from yellow red to brown to chocolate coloured mulberry nodules of variable sizes.

Microscopy

- There are endometrial glands or stroma or both present in endometriotic foci
- In healed endometriosis, fibrous bands and hemosideren laden macrophages are seen.

Locations: Endometriosis occurs in following sites in decreasing order of frequency:

- Ovaries (>60% cases)
- Uterine ligaments
- Rectovaginal septum
- Pouch of Douglas
- Pelvic peritoneum
- Fallopian tubes
- Rectosigmoid colon
- Cervix
- Vagina
- Perineum
- Urinary bladder
- Umbilicus
- Pelvic lymph nodes
- Lungs
- Small intestine
- Kidney
- Bone.

Pathogenesis: There have been certain theories put forward to explain histogenesis of endometriosis which include:

- *Transplantation theory*: The endometrium regurgitates through the fallopian tube and implanted in ectopic sites
- *Multipotential coelomic peritoneal metaplasia theory*: The peritoneal serosa undergoes metaplasia to endometrial stroma in pelvis
- *Induction theory*: Certain substance secreted from endometrium induces the development of endometrial tissue in ectopic sites
- *Vascular or lymphatic dissemination theory*: The endometrial tissue during menses enters blood vessels and lymph channels and is carried to far away places like lungs.

ENDOMETRIAL CARCINOMA

Specific features

- It is the most common gynecological cancer of the female genital tract
- Age group: Seen in 50–70 years of age with median age at presentation is 63 years.

Etiopathogenesis: The risk factors for endometrial cancers include:

- Obesity
- Diabetes mellitus
- Hypertension
- Nulliparity
- Early menarche
- Late menopause
- Patients with ovarian granulosa cell tumors
- Endometrial intraepithelial neoplasia patients
- Cigarette smoking – Reduces risk of endometrial cancer
- Endometrioid endometrial cancers are estrogen dependant; clear cell or serous carcinomas are unassociated with its exposure.

Morphology

Gross morphology (Image B1)

- It presents grossly as
  - Polypoid mass
  - Diffuse infiltrating mass
- Tumors are multifocal with areas of hemorrhage and necrosis.

Microscopy

Based on histological pattern, endometrial carcinoma is of five major types:

- Endometrioid adenocarcinoma (60–80%)
- Endometrioid adenocarcinoma with squamous differentiation (5–7%)
- Serous adenocarcinoma (10–15%)
- Clear cell adenocarcinoma (3–5%)
- Secretory adenocarcinoma
- Adenocarcinomas are of three grades: Well-differentiated, moderately differentiated and poorly differentiated based on the degree of glandular differentiation
- Serous carcinomas are always poorly differentiated and show very poor prognosis.

OVARIAN TUMORS

Specific features

- Ovarian tumors are second most common tumors of female genital tract and account for 5–10% of all female cancers
- Majority of tumors are benign (75–80%) and occurs in 20–50 years age group whereas malignant tumors are seen in 40–70 years.

Etiopathogenesis: Risk factors for ovarian carcinoma include:

- Family history
- Nulliparity
- Gonadal dysgenesis
- OCP usage reduces risk
- Tubal sterilization reduce risk
- Genetic mutations in BRCA 1 and 2 gene, HER-2/neu gene and p53 gene.

Classification (Based on WHO guidelines)

Surface epithelial—stromal tumors

- Serous tumors
    - Benign serous cystadenoma
    - Borderline serous tumor
    - Malignant serous cyst adenocarcinoma
- Mucinous tumors
    - Benign mucinous cystadenoma
    - Borderline mucinous tumor
    - Malignant mucinous cystadenocarcinoma
- Endometrioid tumors
    - Benign
    - Borderline
    - Malignant
- Clear cell tumors
    - Benign
    - Borderline
    - Malignant

Germ cell tumors

- Dysgerminoma
- Yolk sac tumor
- Embryonal carcinoma
- Teratoma
    - Mature
        - Solid
        - Cystic
    - Immature
    - Monodermal
- Mixed germ cell tumors

Sex cord stromal tumors

- Granulosa—stromal cell tumors
    - Granulosa cell tumors
    - Thecoma
    - Fibroma
- Sertoli—stromal cell tumors
    - Androblastoma
    - Sertoli cell tumor
    - Leydig cell tumor
- Steroid cell tumor
- Mixed sex cord stromal tumors.

OVARIAN SURFACE EPITHELIAL TUMORS

Brenner tumor
- They are predominantly unilateral tumors which are composed of dense fibrous stroma and transitional cell rests embedded within it
- They are of three types:
  - Benign
  - Borderline
  - Malignant

Specific features
- They account for >90% of ovarian cancers
- Serous tumors account for 40–50% of surface epithelial tumors
- Serous cystadenocarcinoma are the most common bilateral malignant ovarian tumors.

Histogenesis: Ovarian surface epithelium is transformed into different cell lines to produce tumors:
- Differentiation into fallopian tube epithelium (Serous tumors)
- Differentiation into endocervical mucosa (Mucinous tumors)
- Differentiation into endometrioid mucosa (Endometrioid tumors)
- Differentiation into glycogen rich clear cells of endometrial mucosa (Clear cell tumors)
- Differentiation into mucosa of urinary bladder (Transitional cell tumors).

Serous tumors

Specific features
- They are the most common tumors of ovary accounting for 30–40% of all surface epithelial tumors
- They are most commonly bilateral
- They are of three types:
  - Benign
  - Borderline

  (Benign and Borderline: accounts for 70% of serous tumors)
  - Malignant – account for 25–30% of serous tumors
- Benign and borderline serous tumors occur in 20–50 years age group
- Malignant serous cystadenocarcinoma occur in 40–75 years.

Morphology

Gross morphology
- Benign serous cystadenoma are grossly unicystic with occasional papillary projections and is filled with serous fluid
- Borderline serous tumors have more papillary projections
- Malignant serous cystadenocarcinoma are solid to cystic with multiple papillae and areas of necrosis and hemorrhage. **(Image C1)**

Microscopy
- Microscopically, benign serous cystadenomas show a cyst wall with single layered ciliated tall columnar epithelium **(Fig. 48)**
- Borderline serous tumors show increased papillae which show epithelial stratification, nuclear atypia and increased mitotic activity
- Malignant serous tumors show deep invasion of stroma by tumor cells and they vary from well-differentiated to poorly differentiated. **(Fig. 49)**

OVARIAN SURFACE EPITHELIAL TUMORS (contd.)

Mucinous tumors

Specific features

- They account for 20–30% of ovarian neoplasms
- 70–85% of them are benign tumors whereas rest of them are malignant
- They are of three types:
  - Benign mucinous tumor
  - Borderline mucinous tumor
  - Malignant mucinous cystadenocarcinoma.

Morphology

Benign mucinous tumor

- Grossly, there are large multiloculated cysts filled with sticky gelatinous fluid
- Microscopically, the cysts are lined by mucin secreting tall columnar epithelium with no cillia. **(Fig. 50)**

Borderline mucinous tumor (Image D1)

- Grossly, there are few papillary projections seen in multiloculated cysts
- Microscopically, there is stratification of epithelium with nuclear atypia.

Malignant mucinous cystadenocarcinoma

- Grossly, there are solid areas along with cysts
- Microscopically, there is marked epithelial atypia with stratification and stromal invasion with necrosis and rarely, calcification. **(Fig. 51)**

GERM CELL TUMORS

Definition: They are a heterogenous group of tumors arising from germ cells and have the capacity to differentiate along different cell lines.

Epidemiology

- Germ cell tumors account for 30% of primary ovarian tumors; 95% of which are mature cystic teratoma
- They are malignant in 3% cases
- Malignant germ cell tumors are most common ovarian tumor in children and young adults.

Histogenesis

- When the germ cells undergo neoplastic transformation along trophoblastic lines, it gives rise to choriocarcinoma
- When germ cells stay undifferentiated and undergo neoplastic transformation, it gives rise to dysgerminoma
- When germ cells differentiate into embryonical structures, it gives rise to embryonal carcinoma
- When germ cells differentiate into extraembryonic structures, it gives rise to yolk sac tumor.

Endodermal sinus (Yolk sac) tumor

- It is the second most common germ cell tumor
- Age group: Seen in young adults
- It is characterized by presence of glomeruloid structures called Schiller-Duval bodies.

Dysgerminoma

- It is a tumor composed of monotonous proliferation of germ cells associated with connective tissue septa containing lymphocytes and granuloma
- They are most common malignant germ cell tumors of ovary
- They are seen in 20–30 years of age.

Morphology

Microscopy (Fig. 53)

- They have a monotonous appearance with germ cells having polygonal shape, abundant pale cytoplasm and uniform nuclei
- In between, there are fibrous septae seen containing lymphocytes and granulomata.

Gross morphology: They are well-encapsulated tumors unilateral in 90% cases which are solid uniform grey white to tan in colour. **(Image E1)**

GERM CELL TUMORS (contd.)

Teratoma

- It is a germ cell tumor in which the germ cells differentiate into somatic structures
- Majority of teratomas are biphasic or triphasic.

Types

Mature teratoma

- They are benign tumors commonly called as *dermoid cyst*
- Age group: Most commonly seen in 20–30 years of age
- Grossly, the tumor is a unilocular cyst containing hairs and cheese like sebaceous material with inner surface of cyst wall appearing like crumpled skin **(Image F1)**
- Microscopically, the cyst wall is lined by stratified squamous epithelium with adenexal structures subepithelially **(Fig. 52)**
- 1% of tumors undergo malignant transformation.

Monodermal teratomas

- They contain tissue differentiating along single germ layer
- Most common types are struma ovari and strumal carcinoid.

Immature teratoma

- It is a type of teratoma containing variable amount of immature embryonal tissue structures
- Grossly, the tumor is unilateral, large predominantly solid with few cysts (variegated appearance)
- Microscopically, they are composed of variable amounts of immature embryonal tissue differentiating towards nerves, cartilage, bone and mucous glands etc.

SEX CORD-STROMAL TUMORS

Definition: They are ovarian tumors which originate from primitive sex cords or mesenchymal stroma and are composed of granulosa cells, theca cells, sertoli cells, Leydig cells and fibroblasts singly or in variable compositions.

Epidemiology: They account for 8% of all ovarian tumors.

Types

Leydig cell tumor

Sertoli cell tumor

Granulosa cell tumor

- They are functioning ovarian tumors arising from granulosa cells and seen commonly in postmenopausal women
- They secrete estrogen and inhibin
- They are of two type:
    - Adult type
    - Juvenile type
- Grossly, they are unilateral tumors with grey white to grey yellow areas with focal cysts and hemorrhages
- Microscopically, the tumor cells are polygonal with central coffee bean like nucleus arranged in strands, cords, trabeculae and nodules with formation of call – Exner's bodies which resemble immature follicle.

Fibroma

- They are most common ovarian stromal tumors occurring in all age groups
- Grossly, they are solid grey white
- Microscopically, they are composed of ovarian stromal fibroblasts with variable amounts of collagen.

Thecoma

- They are functioning ovarian tumors of post-menopausal women which are grey white to grey yellow solid tumors
- Microscopically, they are composed of lipid laden theca cells.

GESTATIONAL TROPHOBLASTIC DISEASES

Definition: It is a group of trophoblastic disorders that exhibit proliferation and maturation of trophoblasts along with neoplasm of trophoblastic tissue.

Types

- Hydatidiform mole
  - Complete mole
  - Incomplete mole
  - Invasive mole
- Choriocarcinoma
- Placental site trophoblastic tumor.

Choriocarcinoma

Definition: It is a rapidly invasive widely metastasing malignant neoplasm arising from trophoblasts.

Morphology

- Grossly, it is a fleshy yellow white tumor with extensive ischemic necrosis and hemorrhage
- Microscopically, there is complete absence of abnormal proliferation of cytotrophoblasts, syncytiotrophoblasts and intermediate trophoblasts associated with large areas of hemorrhage.

GESTATIONAL TROPHOBLASTIC DISEASES (contd.)

Hydatidiform mole

Definition: It is a condition in which placenta has grossly swollen chorionic villi resembling bunch of grapes in which there is varying degree of trophoblastic proliferation.

Types

Complete hydatidiform mole

Morphology

- Grossly, molar tissue is voluminous composed of grape like villi; fetal parts are absent **(Image G1)**
- Microscopically, almost all villi show hydropic degeneration which are avascular and show circumferential trophoblastic proliferation. **(Fig. 54)**

Complications

- Patient presents in second trimester of pregnancy with uterine bleeding and large for date uterus
- There is elevation of serum human chorionic gonadotropin levels
- Complications include:
  - Uterine hemorrhage
  - Disseminated intravascular coagulation
  - Uterine perforation
  - Infection
  - Choriocarcinoma (in 2% cases).

Pathogenesis

- It is formed when a sperm with normal DNA fuses with an ovum which has lost its DNA
- The fertilization is followed by duplication of DNA leading to diploid (46, XY) karyotype.

Incomplete (Partial) hydatidiform mole

Pathogenesis

- Partial moles are formed by fusion of two spermatozoa with single ovum containing normal karyotype
- They are triploid or tetraploid.

Morphology

- Grossly, there are variable amount of grape like vesicles seen along with parts of fetus
- Microscopically, there are two populations of chorionic villi seen:
  - Normal viable chorionic villi with central blood vessels
  - Abnormal chorionic villi with hydropic degeneration and avascularity along with variable trophoblastic proliferation
- Malignant transformation is absent.

BENIGN BREAST TUMORS

BENIGN PHYLLODES TUMOR

Definition: It is a tumor characterized by proliferation of intralobular stromal elements accompanied by benign growth of ductal elements.

Morpholo

Gross morphology
- They vary in size from 1 cm to massively enlarged lesions
- The lesions show leafy polypoidal projections in larger lesions.

Microscopy
- There is extensive stromal hyperplasia covered by epithelial cells
- The cellularity and amount of stroma helps in differentiating it from fibroadenoma
- Majority of phyllodes tumor are benign however, malignant counterparts are also seen.

FIBROADENOMA

Definition: It is the most common benign neoplasm of breast composed of epithelial and stromal elements originating from terminal duct lobular unit.

Epidemiology
- Age group: 20–35 years
- They are usually multiple and bilateral
- They enlarge during pregnancy and cease to grow after menopause.

Morphology

Gross morphology (Image H1)
- It is a round, rubbery tumor measuring 2–4 cm in diameter
- Cut surface is glistening grey white.

Micoscopy (Fig. 55)
- They are composed of a mixture of fibrous connective tissue and ducts
- The ducts are of two types—round to oval or compressed ducts which are compressed by surrounding proliferating stroma
- The stroma is delicate, cellular with myxoid areas.

PAPILLOMA

- They are benign tumors located in dilated subareolar ducts
- Grossly, they are few millimetre in diameter
- Microscopically, the epithelium displays papillomatosis with double layered epithelium comprising inner ductal epithelial cells and outer myofibroblasts.

BREAST CARCINOMA

Definition: It is the most common malignancy of breast and one of the most common non skin malignancies in women.

Epidemiology: It is most commonly seen in females >50 years of age and is uncommon before 35 years.

Etiology: Etiological factors include:

- Family history
- Early menarche
- Nulliparity
- Late age at parity
- Infertility
- Lack of breast feeding
- Late age at menopause
- Use of combined oral contraceptives
- Postmenopausal estrogen replacement therapy
- Meat consumption
- Alcohol intake
- Obesity
- Lack of physical activity
- Radiation exposure.

Classification

- *In situ* carcinoma
    - Ductal carcinoma *in situ*
    - Lobular carcinoma *in situ*
- Invasive carcinoma:
    - No special type (NST)
    - Lobular carcinoma
    - Tubular carcinoma
    - Cribriform carcinoma
    - Mucinous (colloid) carcinoma
    - Medullary carcinoma
    - Papillary carcinoma
    - Metaplastic carcinoma.

Pathogenesis

- Mutation in BRCA1 gene on chromosome 17q and BRCA2 gene on chromosome 13q are associated with increased risk of hereditary breast and ovarian malignancies
- Mutations in p53 gene on chromosome 17p are seen in nonhereditary breast carcinoma of women
- Mutations in CHEK2 gene is seen in 5% of women with hereditary breast cancer.

BREAST CARCINOMA (contd.)

Morphology

Gross morphology: The tumors are grey white in color with foci of calcification and irregular margins infiltrating into surrounding breast tissue. **(Image I1)**

Microscopy (Fig. 56)

- The tumor is composed of tumor cells in tubules and solid sheets having varying degree of pleomorphism and mitotic activity
- Higher grade tumor has less number of tubules and high mitotic count
- The tumor is graded by Scarff Bloom-Richardson grading.

Prognosis

- Prognosis is determined by examination of the carcinoma as well as axillary lymph nodes
- The prognostic factors are classified into major and minor prognostic factors.

Minor prognostic factors: These factors are used to determine the women most likely to benefit from chemotherapy and hormone therapy and include:

- Histological type
- Tumor grade
- Estrogen and progesterone receptors
- HER-2/neu expression
- Lymphovascular invasion
- DNA content.

Major prognostic factors

- They are the strongest predictors of death and include:
  - Invasive carcinoma or *in situ* lesion
  - Distant metastasis
  - Lymph node metastasis
  - Tumor size
  - Locally advanced disease
  - Inflammatory carcinoma.

SKIN TUMORS

Basal cell carcinoma

Definition: They are the most common malignant tumors of skin arising from basal cells on sun exposed surfaces.

Etiopathogenesis

- Sun exposure is the most important risk factor
- Nevoid basal cell carcinoma syndrome: It is also seen in association with heritable syndrome in which it is associated with other systemic manifestations
- Germline mutation in PTCH gene on chromosome 9q is responsible for its development.

Morphology

Gross morphology
Grossly, it is of many subtypes:

- Pearly papule with dermal telangiectasia
- Rodent ulcer
- Scaly red sharply demarcated plaque.

Microscopy (Fig. 58): Two patterns of growth are seen:

- *Superficial spreading type* : There are multicentric nests of deeply basophilic epithelial cells having scanty cytoplasm and round to oval nuclei with peripheral palisading radially
- *Nodulocystic type*: The tumor grows more deeply in dermis.

Squamous cell carcinoma

Definition: It is the second most common malignant tumor of skin seen in sun damaged skin of fair individuals.

Etiopathogenesis: The risk factors include:

- Ultraviolet light
- Ionizing radiation
- Chemical carcinogens
- Human papilloma virus
- Mutations in p53 gene are seen in majority of squamous cell carcinomas.

Morphology

Gross morphology

- The lesion is exophytic, grey white mass with or without necrosis.

Microscopy (Fig. 57)

- The tumor cells are present in sheets having abundant eosinophilic cytoplasm and pleomorphic hyperchromatic nuclei
- There are keratin pearls seen in well-differentiated squamous cell carcinomas
- Keratin pearls are whorls of squamous cells with central keratin.

SKIN TUMORS (contd.)

Malignant melanoma

Definition: It is a malignant tumor of skin arising from basal melanocytes.

Etiopathogenesis: The risk factors include:

- Ultraviolet light exposure
- Higher socioeconomic status
- Lightly pigmented individuals
- Mutations in p16 INK4a gene on chromosome 9p is seen in familial cases of malignant melanoma.

Prognosis: The melanomas which are <1.7 mm thick with no evident mitosis and exhibiting lymphocytic infiltrate rarely metastasize whereas melanomas with >3.6 mm depth, >6 mitoses/mm^2 and without lymphocytic infiltrate frequently metastasize and have poor prognosis.

Morphology

Gross morphology: The lesion is elevated, dark brown >1 cm in diameter with or without ulceration.

Microscopy (Fig. 59)

- The tumors has radial and vertical growth phase
- Individual melanoma cells have moderate eosinophilic cytoplasm and large nuclei with irregular contours; have clumped chromatin at periphery of nuclear membrane and eosinophilic prominent nucleoli with variable amount of melanin.

THYROIDITIS

Definition: It is a heterogenous group of inflammatory disorders of thyroid gland caused by autoimmune or infectious etiology.

Types

Infectious thyroiditis

Subacute granulomatous thyroiditis
- Also known as de Quervain or giant cell thyroiditis
- It is an infrequent self-limiting granulomatous inflammation of thyroid which occurs secondary to viral upper respiratory tract infections, e.g. influenza, adenovirus, echovirus and coxsackievirus
- F >M; 30–50 years age group.

Morphology

Gross morphology
- Thyroid is enlarged with cut surface showing firm, pale white areas.

Microscopy
- Patchy destruction of thyroid follicles with release of colloid
- There is inflammatory infiltrate composed of lymphocytes, plasma cells, macrophages and foreign body type multinucleated giant cells
- Inflammation is followed by fibrosis.

Autoimmune thyroiditis

Subacute lymphocytic thyroiditis
- Also known as *silent thyroiditis*
- It is characterized by painless enlargement of thyroid; self-limiting hyperthyroidism and destruction of thyroid parenchyma by lymphocytes
- It is most common in middle aged females predominantly in postpartum period.

Morphology

Microscopy: There is patchy disruption of thyroid follicles with formation of lymphoid germinal centres.

Gross morphology: The thyroid gland is mildly enlarged with normal cut surface.

Autoimmune thyroiditis (contd.)

Hashimoto thyroiditis

- **Definition:** It is characterized by presence of circulating antibodies to thyroid antigens and features of cell mediated immunity to thyroid tissue
- Age – 40–50 years; F >M

Morphology

Gross morphology

- The thyroid gland is diffusely enlarged and firm with pale tan and fleshy cut surface resembling a lymph node.

Microscopy

- Atrophy and destruction of thyroid follicles
- Hurthle cell or Askanazy cell change of follicular epithelial cells
- Diffuse infiltrate of lymphocytes and plasma cells in interstitial tissue
- Rarely, there is transformation to non-Hodgkin lymphoma.

Pathogenesis

- It is an autoimmune disease involving both cellular and hormonal immunity.
- The thyroid antigens lead to activation of CD4 + T-cells which in turn activate CD8 + T-cells which attack thyroid epithelial cells
- Thyroid cells also express major histocompatibility complex class II molecules which activate T-cells to produce interferons for expansion of CD8 + T-cell population
- Activated CD4 + T-cells recruit B-lymphocytes that produce antibodies againt thyroid microsomal peroxidase, thyroglobulin and thyroid stimulating hormone receptor.

GOITRE

Definition: It is the enlargement of thyroid gland which reflects decreased production of thyroxine.

Types

Multinodular goitre

Definition: It refers to irregular enlargement of thyroid gland with formation of multiple nodules.

Morphology

Microscopy

- There are variably sized thyroid follicles seen filled with colloid and lined by flattened follicular epithelial cells
- Variable amount of calcification, fibrosis and hemorrhage seen.

Gross morphology (Image J1)

- They thyroid gland is asymmetrically enlarged with formation of multiple nodules
- Cut surface show irregular large nodules filled with colloid and show degenerative change like fibrosis, hemorrhage and calcification.

Diffuse non-toxic goitre

Definition: It refers to diffuse enlargement of thyroid gland with no nodule formation

- F : M ratio is 8 : 1
- Age group: Adolescence and pregnancy.

Types

Endemic goitre

- It occurs in locations where soil contains low level of iodine
- It is more common than sporadic goiter
- It is also seen in places where goitrogens are eaten in excess.

Sporadic goiter

- It is less common to endemic goitre
- Causes include improper thyroxine synthesis due to various causes.

Morphology

Gross morphology

The thyroid gland is diffusely and symmetrically enlarged and weighs 100–150 gm.

Microscopy: There are two phases:

- *Hyperplastic phase*: In this phase, follicles are small lined by tall columnar epithelium with scanty colloid.
- *Involution phase*: In this phase, follicles are large lined by flattened epithelium and filled with abundant colloid. **(Fig. 60)**

THYROID NEOPLASMS

Benign thyroid tumors

Follicular adenoma

Definition: It is a benign neoplasm of thyroid that exhibits follicular differentiation and is the most common tumor of thyroid.

Morphology

Gross morphology

- They are solitary, well-circumscribed nodules 1–3 cm in diameter which protrudes from surface of thyroid
- The cut surface of tumor is soft and paler than surrounding stroma.

Microscopy

- There are uniform colloid filled follicles seen which are different from the follicles outside
- The follicular cells do not invade the capsule a feature differentiating it from follicular carcinoma
- Variants of follicular adenoma are:
  - Simple adenoma
  - Colloid adenoma
  - Hurthle cell adenoma
  - Atypical adenoma
  - Trabecular adenoma.

Malignant thyroid tumors

Follicular carcinoma of thyroid

- It is second most common malignant tumor of thyroid and is purely follicular with no papillary areas
- Age group: >40 years
- Sex: F : M : : 3 : 11
- Nodular goiter predisposes it.

Pathogenesis

- N—RAS mutation is seen in >50% of follicular thyroid carcinomas
- PAX 8—PPARγ1 fusion gene due to translocation t (2, 3) is seen in 30–40% cases.

Morphology

Microscopy

- The tumor shows variably sized follicles which are distinct from surrounding thyroid tissue
- There is capsular invasion noted by the tumor follicles.

Gross morphology

- The tumor is 3–6 cm encapsulated lesion with presence of capsular invasion
- Cut surface is fleshy and solid.

Malignant thyroid tumors (contd.)

Papillary carcinoma of thyroid

- They are the most common cancer of thyroid
- Age group: 20–50 years
- Sex: F: M : : 3:1

Pathogenesis

- Risk factors seen in association with it are:
  - Iodine excess
  - External radiation exposure in head and neck region
  - *Genetic factors*: It is 4–10 times more common in first degree relatives of patients with papillary thyroid carcinoma
  - *Somatic mutations*: RET proto-oncogene mutations on chromosome 10q11.2 are common in papillary thyroid carcinoma.

Morphology

Gross morphology

- They are solitary to multiple, pale, firm to hard, gritty lesions
- They can be encapsulated or show infiltrative margins
- Cut surface shows papillae.

Microscopy (Fig. 61)

- There are branching papillae seen lined by single or stratified layer of cuboidal to columnar cells and a fibrovascular core
- The lining neoplastic cells show crowding with overlapping of nucleus
- The nuclei are clear in majority of them (Orphan–Annie eye or ground glass appearance) with few showing eosinophilic pseudoinlusions and nuclear grooves
- Calcospherites called as *Psammoma bodies* are seen in core of papillae in > 50% cases
- Capsular and lymphovascular invasion is classically seen.

DIABETES MELLITUS

Definition: It is a group of metabolic disorder showing a common finding of hyperglycemia.

Classification

Type II or non-insulin dependent diabetes mellitus (NIDDM)

Pathogenesis

- *Genetic factors*:
  - 60–70% of patients have a parent or sibling with this disease
  - 95–100% of monozygotic twins have the disease
- *Glucose metabolism*:
  - Discordance between insulin and glucagon levels lead to altered glucose metabolism causing hyperglycemia
- *β-cell dysfunction*:
  - There is impaired β-cell insulin release in response to hyperglycemia
  - Maturity onset diabetes of young (MODY) occurs due to mutation in glucokinase enzyme
- Obesity and insulin resistance are closely related as adipocytes release tumor necrosis factor and adiponectin that reduce peripheral insulin sensitivity.

Definition: It is a hetrogenous disorder characterized by reduced sensitivity to insulin and impaired insulin secretion.

Morphology

- There is very mild reduction in islet cell mass
- Amyloid replacement of islets appear as pink amorphous material.

Type I or insulin dependent diabetes mellitus

Morphology

- Reduction in number and size of islets
- Lymphocytic infiltration of islets is noted.

Definition: It is a lifelong disorder of glucose homeostasis that results from autoimmune destruction of β-cells of islets of Langerhans.

Pathogenesis

- *Genetic factors*:
  - Less than 20% patients have sibling or parent with disease
  - It is seen in <50% of identical twins
  - 90% of IDDM patients show HLADR3 or HLADR4 or both as compared to general population
- *Autoimmunity*: Mechanisms postulated as causing autoimmune destruction of β-cells are:
  - CD 8 + T-cells kill β-cells directly and secrete cytokines to activate macrophages
  - Locally produced cytokines interferon γ by T-cells and tumor necrosis factor, interleukin 1 by macrophages damage β-cells
  - Autoantibodies against islet cells and insulin are seen in blood of 70–80% patients
- *Environmental factors*:
  - Infections by rubella and coxsackie B virus induce autoimmune destruction of β-cells Langhans.

COMPLICATIONS OF DIABETES MELLITUS

Classification

Vascular complications

Macrovascular disease
- Atherosclerosis leading to:
    - Peripheral vascular disease
    - Myocardial infarction
    - Cerebrovascular hemorrhage.

Microvascular disease
- Retinopathy
- Nephropathy.

Neurological complication
- Peripheral neuropathy
- Autonomic neuropathy.

Ocular complication
- Glaucoma
- Cataract
- Retinopathy.

Infections

Metabolic complications
- Diabetic ketoacidosis
- Hyperosmolar non-ketotic coma.

Hyperosmolar nonketotic coma
- It is more common in type II diabetes mellitus
- It is seen due to severe dehydration resulting from osmotic diuresis in patients who do not drink water to compensate it.

Diabetic ketoacidosis
- It is a serious complication most commonly seen in type I diabetes mellitus but also is seen in type II diabetes mellitus
- Insulin deficiency stimulates lipoprotein lipase leading to increased level of free fatty acids; these fee fatty acids are esterfied to acyl coenzyme A and oxidized in hepatocyte mitochondria to produce ketone bodies.

Pathogenesis: Variety of biochemical mechanisms have been proposed:
- *Protein glycosylation*: Glucose binds non-enzymatically with proteins giving rise to advanced glycosylation end products (AGE) which produce cross- linkage between various extracellular matrix protein leading to decreased elasticity of tissues
- *Sorbitol pathway*: Hyperglycemia leads to excessive uptake of glucose by tissues which is metabolized by tissue reductase to sorbitol which accumulates in nerves, retina, lens and kidney leading to tissue injury
- *Protein kinase C activation*: Hyper-glycemia induces activation of protein kinase C which induces following effects:
    - Increased provasculogenic factors → Neovascularization → Diabetic retinopathy
    - Increased production of procoagulant molecule plasminogen activator inhibitor I molecule (PAI 1) leading to vaso-occlusive episodes.

Diabetic nephropathy
- Second most common cause of death after myocardial infarction
- The lesions seen are:
    - Glomerular lesions – capillary basement membrane thickening, diffuse mesangial sclerosis and nodular glomerulosclerosis
    - Renal arteriosclerosis
    - Pyelonephritis with or without necrotizing papillitis.

MULTIPLE ENDOCRINE NEOPLASIA SYNDROMES

Definition: They are a group of genetically inherited diseases resulting in hyperplasia, adenomas and carcinomas of multiple endocrine organs.

Etiopathogenesis

- MEN 1 syndrome is caused by germline mutation in MEN 1 gene located at chromosome 11q13
- MEN 2 syndrome is caused by germline mutation in RET gene located at chromosome 10q11.2.

Types

MEN type 1

- It is also known as *Wermer's syndrome*
- It causes abnormalities in parathyroid, pancreas and pituitary glands
- The lesions include:
  - Primary hyperparathyroidism due to parathyroid hyperplasia
  - Pancreatic benign or malignant endocrine tumors
  - Pituitary prolactinomas.

MEN type 2

Subtypes

MEN type 2A

- It is also known as *Sipple syndrome*
- It causes abnormalities in adrenal medulla, thyroid and parathyroid
- The lesions include:
  - Parathyroid hyperplasia
  - Pheochromocytoma
  - Medullary carcinoma of thyroid.

Familial medullary thyroid cancer

- It is characterized by medullary carcinoma of thyroid but without any other abnormality.

MEN type 2B

- It is characterized by following abnormalities:
  - Medullary thyroid carcinoma
  - Pheochromocytoma
  - Neuromas or ganglioneuromas in skin, eye, respiratory tract and gastrointestinal tract
  - Marfanoid habitus.

OSTEOMYELITIS

Definition: It is defined as inflammation of bone and bone marrow as a complication of systemic infections.

Types

Tuberculous osteomyelitis

- It is more common in third world countries.
- It is seen in adolescent and young adults.
- The bacteria reach bone by hematogenous route, direct extension from tracheobronchial tree or via draining lymphatics into the rib or vertebrae.

Morphology

Gross morphology

- Most common site of involvement is spine; predominantly the dorsal and lumbar vertebrae
- Tuberculosis of spine is called as *Pott disease*
- The next most common sites of involvement are knee and hip.

Microscopy

- Dead necrotic bone called *sequestrum* is seen
- There is caseous necrosis along with epithelioid cell granulomata seen in the underlying subperiosteal region.

Types (contd.)

Pyogenic osteomyelitis

- It is defined as inflammation of bone and bone marrow caused by pyogenic bacteria.

Pathogenesis

- Infectious organism reaches bone by direct penetration or hematogenous spread
- The infection affects the metaphysic of bone due to unique blood supply. The blood vessels form a loop into the calcified plate and return back to medullary cavity due to which blood supply is slow in this region
- This facilitates penetration of organism from blood vessels to extravascular matrix where it proliferates to cause pressure on vessel loop leading to vascular compromise and bone necrosis
- The pus and bacteria, then, extend into endosteal vascular channels that supply cortex and thus, subperiosteally which breaks and releases into surrounding soft tissue (sequestrum) and skin forming sinus
- The reactive new bone forms to contain the infection (involucrum).

Etiology

- The most common microbes causing it are:
  - *Staphylococus aureus (70–90%)*
  - *Escherichia coli*
  - *Neisseria gonorrhea*
  - *Hemophilus influenzae*
  - *Salmonella typhi.*

Morphology

Microscopy (Fig. 62)

- The dead necrotic bone is called *sequestrum*
- The reactive woven bone forms to contain the infection and is called as involucrum.

Gross morphology

- The morphological changes depend on whether the inection is acute, subacute and chronic
- The abscesses in subperiosteal region lead to ischemic necrosis of overlying bone that is released into surrounding tissue and forms a sinus tract.

Specialized variants

- *Brodie abscess*: It consists of reactive woven bone of periosteum and endosteum to contain infection
- *Scleroring osteomyelitis of Garre*: It develops in the jaw associated with extensive new bone formation that obscures underlying bone structures.

CLASSIFICATION OF BONE TUMORS

Hematopoeitic tumors
- Malignant: Multiple myeloma, malignant lymphoma.

Chondrogenic (cartilage forming) tumors
- Benign: Osteochondroma, chondroma, chondroblastoma, chondromyxoid fibroma
- Malignant: Chondrosarcoma.

Osteogenic (bone forming) tumors
- Benign: Osteoid osteoma, osteoblastoma
- Malignant: Osteosarcoma.

Lipogenic tumors
- Benign: Lipoma
- Malignant: Liposarcoma.

Fibrogenic tumors
- Benign: Desmoplastic fibroma
- Malignant: Fibrosarcoma

Fibrohistiocytic tumors
- Benign: Benign fibrous histiocytoma
- Malignant: Malignant fibrous histiocytoma.

Vascular tumors
- Benign: Hemangioma
- Malignant: Hemangioendothelioma, hemangiopericytoma.

Notochordal tumors
- Malignant: Chordoma

Neurogenic tumors
- Benign: Neurilemmoma

Tumors of unknown origin
- Benign: Osteoclastoma
- Malignant: Malignant giant cell tumor, Ewing sarcoma, adamantinoma.

OSTEOSARCOMA

Definition: It is a highly malignant bone tumor characterized by formation of bone matrix by tumor cells
- It is also known as *osteogenic sarcoma*.

Epidemiology
- It comprises one-fifth of all bone tumors
- It is the most common primary malignant tumor of bone exclusive of lymphoma and multiple myeloma
- Age group: It is most common in 10–20 years of age
- Sex: M : F : : 2 : 1

Clinicoradiological features
- They clinically present as painful enlarging masses associated with fever
- X-ray findings: Codman triangle classically seen which is formed due to elevation of periosteum away from the cortex.

Pathogenesis
- Two-thirds cases of osteosarcoma show mutations in retinoblastoma gene and many tumors contain p53 gene mutation
- Osteosarcomas are of 2 types:
  - *Primary osteosarcoma*: When there is no underlying previous bone pathology
  - *Secondary osteosarcoma*: When it develops in patients with Paget disease or post-exposure to radiation.

Locations
- The tumor arises from metaphysis of bone
- 60% are located around knee joint
- Flat bones are involved in patients >25 years of age.

Morphology

Gross morphology (Image K1)
Grossly, they are bulky tumors which are gritty, grey white and contains areas of hemorrhage and cystic degeneration.

Microscopic features (Fig. 63)
- Histologically, tumor cells are pleomorphic and display osteoblastic differentiation producing woven bone (malignant osteoid) which has coarse, lace like architecture
- Histological subtypes:
  - Osteoblastic variant
  - Chondroblastic variant
  - Fibroblastic variant
  - Telangiectatic variant
  - Small cell variant
  - Giant cell variant.

EWING SARCOMA

Definition: It is an uncommon malignant bone tumor composed of uniform small round cells having unknown origin.

Epidemiology

- It comprises 5% of all bone tumors
- Age group affected: 5–10 years
- Sex: Males are affected twice as commonly as females
- They are second most common childhood bone sarcomas after osteosarcoma.

Pathogenesis

- It is thought to arise from primitive marrow elements or immature mesenchyme
- 90% of these tumors show translocation t (11, 22) which results in a fusion gene EWS-FLI1.

Clinicoradiological findings

- The patient presents with painful enlarging masses associated with or without fever
- X-ray findings: X-ray shows a destructive, lytic lesion that has invasive margins with characteristic periosteal reaction giving an *onionskin appearance.*

Locations

- The tumor arises from diaphysis of long tubular bones especially femur, humerus and tibia
- Flat bones of pelvis are also involved.

Morphology

Gross morphology

- It is soft and greyish white studded by foci of hemorrhage and necrosis
- The tumor may invade the medullary cavity or the soft tissue around the cortex of bone.

Microscopic features (Fig. 64)

- The tumor cells appear as sheets of closely packed small round cells with little cytoplasm containing glycogen and are up to twice the size of lymphocytes
- The fibrous bands separate the sheet of cells into irregular nests
- Mitoses are infrequent.

GIANT CELL TUMOR (OSTEOCLASTOMA)

Definition: It is a locally aggressive potentially malignant neoplasm characterized by presence of osteoclastic multinucleated giant cells randomly and uniformly distributed in the background of proliferating mononuclear cells.

Epidemiology

- They represent 4–5% of all primary bone tumors
- It is more common in Asians as compared to Western countries
- Age group: 20 to 45 years
- Sex: Females are slightly more affected than males.

Locations

- The tumor arises from metaphysic and epiphysis
- Most common locations are ends of long bones: Distal femur, proximal tibia, distal radius and proximal humerus
- In 5% cases, it involves flat bones, most common being sacrum.

Clinicoradiological findings

- The patient presents with pain, swelling and restricted joint movement
- X-ray findings: X-ray shows a lytic lesion with sclerotic margins sometimes with trabeculated *soap bubble appearance.*

Morphology

Gross morphology

- The tumor is clearly circumscribed with light brown and soft cut surface
- Numerous hemorrhagic and necrotic areas may be seen
- Aggressive tumors penetrate the bone cortex into the surrounding soft tissue.

Microscopic features

- The tumor is composed of sheets of uniform oval mononuclear cells with syncytial growth pattern
- There are numerous osteoclast like giant cells seen with 50–100 nuclei
- There is variable amount of mitoses seen.

OSTEOPOROSIS

Definition: It is a metabolic bone disease characterized by diffuse skeletal lesions in which normally mineralized bone is decreased in mass to the point that it no longer provides adequate mechanical support.

Epidemiology

- It commonly occurs in 5th or 6th decade of life onwards
- It is more common in white population as compared to blacks
- Females are affected twice as common to males.

Etiology: It is classified into two categories:

- *Primary osteoporosis*: It is further subclassified into 2 types:
    - Type I primary osteoporosis: It occurs principally in post-menopausal women
    - Type II primary osteoporosis: It is seen in both sexes in old age.
- *Secondary osteoporosis*:
    - Endocrine disorder Hyper-parathyroidism, hypogonadism, pituitary adenoma, type I diabetes mellitus, Addison disease
    - Neoplasm: Multiple myeloma, bone metastatic carcinoma
    - Gastrointestinal: Vitamin C and D deficiency, hepatic insufficiency, malabsorption
    - Drugs: Alcohol, corticosteroids, anticoagulants, anticonvulsants
    - Miscellaneous: Immobilization, homocysteinemia, anemia.

Morphology

Gross morphology

- It affects all bones of body, but, majority affects weight bearing bones which include vertebral bodies and neck of femur.

Microscopy

- The affected bone show decreased total mass and thinning of bony cortex and trabeculae with widening of Haversian canals.

Pathogenesis

- Type I primary osteoporosis is due to an increase in osteoclast activity
- Type II primary osteoporosis is due to attenuated osteoblast function which are unable to replace the bone removed during resorptive phase of remodeling cycle
- Factors affecting osteoporosis include:
    - *Genetic factors*: The risk of osteoporosis is high in persons with low peak bone mass; the peak bone mass is lower in women as compared to men and whites or Asians as compared to blacks
    - *Physical activity*: Decreased physical activity leads to accelerated bone resorption
    - *Calcium absorption and vitamin D*: Absorption of calcium decreases with age; there is low circulating level of 1, 25 $(OH)_2$ D in persons with osteoporosis.

OSTEOARTHRITIS

Definition: It is a degenerative articular joint disease that is characterized by a slowly progressive destruction of articular cartilage that is manifested in weight bearing joints and fingers of older persons or joints of younger persons subjected to trauma.

Epidemiology

- It is commonly seen in old age; 85% of persons aged between 75–80 are affected
- In patients <45 years, males are affected commonly to females; in patients >55 years, females are affected more than males.

Etiopathogenesis: Factors playing major role in osteoarthritis are:

- *Increased unit load*: Abnormal force on articular cartilage results in death of chondrocytes leading to its degradation
- *Resilience of articular cartilage*: It is lost in old age due to excess of water bonding with it
- *Stiffness of subchondral coarse cancellous bone*: Microfractures formed in cancellous bone due to stiffness leads to increase pressure on articular cartilage
- *Biochemical abnormalitites*: Proteoglycan content and aggregation decrease; chain length of glycosa minoglycans decreases; collagen bands are thicker than normal and water content of cartilage increases; synthesis of cartilage matrix and number of chondrocytes decreases with advanced disease.

Morphology

Gross morphology

- The articular cartilage show fibrillations and is sloughed
- The synovium is congested and fibrotic
- The exposed bones give an ivory like appearance.

Microscopy

- Initially, there is decreased metachromatic staining due to loss of proteoglycans
- The lacunae of cartilage are empty due to death of chondrocytes
- There are fibrillations produced on cartilage
- Cartilage fragments and lodge into synovium causing hyperemia, hypertrophy and induce inflammation
- New blood vessels enter from subchondral bone into cracks in cartilage and induce osteoclastic resorption
- The subchondral bone is burnished and eventually cracks and are filled with synovial fluid forming subchondral bone cysts
- Osteophytes are developed in lateral surface of joint where mesenchymal tissue of synovium modulates into osteoblasts and chondroblasts to form cartilage and bone
- Osteophytes in fingers are called *Heberden nodes*.

Radiological features

- Joints affected are proximal and distal interphalyngeal joints of hands, knee, hip, cervical and lumbar spine
- The joint space is narrowed due to loss of articular cartilage
- Increased thickness of subchondral bone
- Subchondral bone cysts
- Large peripheral growth of cartilage and bone called *osteophytes seen.*

RHEUMATOID ARTHRITIS

Definition: It is a systemic chronic inflammatory disorder that affects multiple tissues and organs principally the joints producing a nonsuppurative, proliferative and inflammatory synovitis leading to destruction of articular cartilage and ankylosis of joints.

Epidemiology
- Age group affected: 4th to 7th decade
- Women are affected thrice as common to men.

Etiopathogenesis
- It is an autoimmune disease triggered by exposure of unknown antigen in a genetically susceptible lost.
- Factors implicated in development of rheumatoid arthritis are:
  - *Genetic factors*: There is increased incidence in monozygotic twins and first degree relatives; associated with HLA – DRB1 gene
  - *Humoral immunity*: Rheumatoid factor which is an autoantibody formed against Fc fragment of IgG and is an IgM molecule in majority of the cases
  - *Cellular immunity*: CD4 + helper T- cells accumulate at site and activate macrophages that release cytokines leading to pannus formation.
  - *Local factors*: Synoviocytes of patients exhibits decreased response to glucocorticoids and increased production of hyaluronate.

Morphology

Microscopy
- Pannus formation occurs in synovium composed of a mass of synoviocytes and synovial stroma along with inflammatory cells, granulation tissue and fibroblasts
- It causes erosion of articular cartilage leading to bony ankylosis
- Rheumatoid nodule shows central fibrinoid necrosis palisaded by epithelioid histiocytes, lymphocytes and plasma cells.

Gross morphology
- The articular joints which are majorly affected are proximal interphalangeal joints, metacarpophalangeal joints, elbow, knee, ankle and spine
- The synovium is edematous, thickened and hyperplastic transforming its smooth contour into bulbuous fronds
- Rheumatoid nodules are firm tender subcutaneous nodules occurring on ulnar aspect of forearms, elbows, occiput and lumbosacral area.

GOUT

Definition: It is a heterogenous group of diseases in which the common denominator is an increased serum uric acid level and deposition of urate crystals in joints and kidneys.

Classification

- *Primary gout*: Hyperuricemia in absence of any other disease
- Secondary gout: Hyperuricemia associated with other conditions like leukemia, chronic renal diseases and Lesch-Nyhan syndrome.

Etiology: The risk factors include:

- Age: >30 years of age
- Genetic predisposition
- Heavy alcohol consumption
- Obesity
- Drugs e.g. thiazide diuretics
- Lead toxicity.

Pathogenesis

- The major pathogenic change is precipitation of monosodium urate crystals in joints
- Serum uric acid level >7 mg/dl leads to accumulation of urate crystals in joints
- Hyperuricemia results from:
  - Overproduction of purines
  - Increased catabolism of uric acid
  - Decreased salvage of free purine bases
  - Decreased urinary excretion of uric acid.

Morphology

- The distinctive changes in gout are:
  - Acute arthritis
  - Chronic tophaceous arthritis
  - Tophi in various locations
  - Gouty nephropathy.

Acute arthritis: Characterized by

- Dense neutrophilic infiltrate in synovium and synovial fluid.
- There are long needle shaped, negatively birefringent monosodium urate crystals seen in synovial fluid or neutrophils.

Gouty nephropathy

- Deposition of monosodium urate in renal medullary interstitium
- Intratubular uric acid precipitation leads to urate calculi.

Tophi in various locations

- Tophi are deposited in
  - Articular cartilage
  - Ligaments
  - Tendens
  - Bursae around joints
  - Achilles tendon
  - Ear lobes
  - Nasal cartilage
  - Skin of fingertips, palms and soles.

Chronic tophaceous gout

- Tophi are large aggregates of urate crystals surrounded by intense inflammation comprising lymphocytes, histiocytes and foreign body type of giant cells.
- The synovium is hyperplastic, fibrotic with inflammatory cells.

MENINGITIS

Definition: It is defined as an inflammatory process of leptomeninges and CSF within the subarachnoid space.

Classification: It is classified into two groups:

a. *Acute meningitis*
   - Acute pyogenic meningitis
   - Acute aseptic meningitis

b. *Chronic meningitis*
   - Chronic tubercular meningitis
   - Chronic spirochaetal meningitis
   - Chronic cryptococcal meningitis.

Acute viral meningitis

Morphology
- No distinctive morphological changes except brain swelling.

CSF findings
- Moderate increase in CSF protein
- Near normal CSF glucose
- CSF cytology: Lymphocytic leucocytosis
- Mildly increased CSF pressure.

Etiopathogenesis
- In 70% cases, viruses are detected which include:
  - Enterovirus
  - Echovirus
  - Coxsackievirus
  - Poliovirus.

Acute pyogenic meningitis

CSF findings
- Increased CSF pressure
- Increased CSF protein
- Decreased CSF glucose
- CSF cell count: Elevated up to 1 lakh cells/μl.

Morphology
- The CSF is cloudy and frankly purulent
- There is exudates on the brain surface beneath the meninges
- The meningeal blood vessels are congested
- Microscopically, neutrophils fill the entire subarachnoid space.

Etiopathogenesis
- In neonates, the most common organisms include *E. coli* and group B *Streptococcus.*
- In old age, most common organisms include *Streptococcus pneumonia* and *Listeria monocytogenes.*
- In young adults, *Neisseria meningitidis* is most common bacteria causing meningitis.

Chronic tubercular meningitis

CSF findings
- Increased CSF pressure
- Increased CSF protein
- Normal or mildly decreased CSF glucose
- Mixed CSF leucocytosis composed of mononuclear cells or mixture of mononuclear cells and neutrophils.

Morphology
- Grossly, subarachnoid space contains gelatinous or fibrinous exudates mostly at base of brain
- The CSF shows a cob web coagulum on standing
- Microscopically, epithelioid cell granulomas, lymphocyte, plasma cells and macrophages are seen.

CENTRAL NERVOUS SYSTEM (CNS) TUMORS

Specific features

- They comprise 20% of all cancers of childhood
- 70% of CNS tumors arise in posterior fossa
- Characteristic features of CNS tumors:
  - Distinction between benign and malignant tumors is less evident
  - Primary tumors of CNS rarely metastasize outside CNS
  - Anatomical location of tumor leads to lethal consequences irrespective of histological classification.

Classification: Based on the origin

- Gliomas: Originate from neuroectoderm
- Neuronal tumors
- Meningiomas
- Poorly differentiated neoplasms
- Metastatic tumors.

GLIOMAS

Astrocytoma

Definition: They are gliomas composed of well-differentiated astrocytes.

Epidemiology: It comprises 20% of primary intracranial neoplasms.

Morphology

Gross morphology

- Astrocytomas are most frequently located in cerebral hemisphere in adults, optic nerve, wall of third ventricle, midbrain pons and cerebellum
- The tumor varies in size from few centimetres to enormous size
- Cut surface of the tumor is soft or firm, gelatinous with cystic degeneration.

Microscopy

- The tumor is composed of variable amount of glial cells with cytoplasmic processes and round nuclei
- The astrocytoma variants are:
  - Fibrillary astrocytoma
  - Gemistocytic astrocytoma
  - Pilocytic astrocytoma.

Oligodendroglioma

Definition: They are gliomas composed of oligodendrocytes.

Epidemiology

- The tumor constitutes 5–15% of gliomas
- They are most common in 4th and 5th decades of life.

Morphology

Gross morphology

- They are most commonly seen in white matter of cerebral hemispheres
- Grossly, they are well-circumscribed, gelatinous, grey colored masses
- Calcification varying in amount is seen in 80–95% of tumors.

Microscopy

- The tumor is composed of sheets of regular cells with round nucleus, finely granular chromatin and clear cytoplasm
- Mitotic activity is scarce
- Calcification is seen in 80% cases
- There are many anastomosing capillaries seen.

GLIOMAS (contd.)

Ependymoma

Definition: They are the gliomas arising from ependymal lining of the ventricular cavities.

Epidemiology: They account for 5–10% cases.

Morphology

Microscopy

- They are composed of cells with round to oval nuclei with abundant granular chromatin
- Tumor cells form rosettes and canals with long delicate processes extending into the lumen
- Perivascular pseudorosettes are also seen.

Gross morphology

- In children, the tumor is located in 4th ventricle, however, in adults, it is most commonly seen in spinal cord
- The ventricular tumor is solid to papillary masses, whereas spinal tumors are predominantly solid masses.

MENINGIOMA

Definition: They are tumors arising from meningothelial cells of arachnoid.

Epidemiology
- They account for 20–25% of tumors of CNS
- They are most common intracranial neoplasm
- They are predominantly benign; rarely malignant.

Etiopathogenesis
- Deletion of chromosome 22q12 leading to loss of NF2 tumor suppressor gene.

Morphology

Gross morphology (Image L1)
- The are round, bosselated, or lobulated well-demarcated dural-based nodules impinging on surrounding brain parenchyma but can be easily separated from it
- Cut section is usually homogenous to granular; cystic degeneration and hemorrhages
are not seen; necrosis may be seen in high grade tumors
- En plaque variant: Certain tumors have carpet like growth pattern along the dura.

Microscopy
- They are histologically graded I–III according to WHO grading system

- WHO grade I/IV tumors:
  - Syncytial, fibroblastic, transitional, Psammomatous, angiomatous, secretory and microcystic variant are grade I
  - In syncytial variant, whorls of meningothelial cells are seen in clusters **(Fig. 66)**
  - In fibroblastic variant, elongated cells with abundant collagen seen
  - In transitional variant, combination of syncytial and fibroblastic variants seen

- WHO grade II/IV(atypical) tumors:
  - >4 mitoses/10hpf, sheeting architecture, small rounded cells, macronucleoli, hypercellularity, necrosis, and brain invasion are criteria for diagnosis
  - Includes chordoid and clear cell variant.

- WHO grade III/IV(anaplastic) tumors:
  - >20 mitoses/10 hpf and frank anaplasia are criteria for diagnosis
  - Includes papillary and rhabdoid variant.

Index